# Restoring Psychotherapy as the First Line Intervention in Behavioral Care

D1508655

Nicholas A. Cummings, Ph.D., Sc.D.

and William O'Donohue, Ph.D.

Editors

# IP

## ITHACA PRESS

NEW YORK

Ithaca Press
3 Kimberly Drive, Suite B
Dryden, New York 13053 USA
www.IthacaPress.com

Copyright © 2012 Nicholas Cummings
*Restoring Psychotherapy as the First Line Intervention in Behavioral Care*

*All rights reserved under International and
Pan American Copyright Law, including the
right of reproduction in whole or in part,
without the written permission of the publisher.
Requests for such permission should be addressed to
Ithaca Press, 3 Kimberly Drive, Suite B, Dryden,
New York 13053 USA*

Cover Design     Gary Hoffman
Book Design      Gary Hoffman

Manufactured in the United States of America

9  8  7  6  5  4  3  2  1

Library of Congress Cataloging-in-Data Available

First Edition

Printed in the United States of America

**ISBN  978-0-9839121-1-8**

www.Prescient Books.com
www.DrNicholasCummings.com

# Prologue

"Restoring Psychotherapy as the First Line Intervention in Behavioral Health" is the title of a prescient and provocative conference held on March 18–19, 2011 in the Downtown Campus of Arizona State University (ASU). Co-sponsored by ASU's Nicholas A. Cummings Doctor of Behavioral Health Program (www.dbh.asu.edu) and the Cummings Foundation for Behavioral Health (www.thecummingsfoundation.org), the conference addressed the so-called "medicalization" of mental health that resulted in the disruption of psychotherapy by psychotropic medication, as well as the attendant difficulties that have ensued.

This conference featured renown authorities from as far away as the United Kingdom, each of whom addressed particular aspects of this disruption, all leading toward restoring psychotherapy to its rightful importance. The presenters gave freely of their time in anticipation that their contribution will comprise a book of which 3000 copies will be distributed by the Cummings Foundation to the nation's mental healthcare leaders and to the Members of the Congress of the United States. If you are receiving this book it is on that basis.

Inquiries should be directed to Linda Goddard, Executive Assistant, Cummings Foundation for Behavioral Health, 4781 Caughlin Parkway, Reno, Nevada 89519.

Thank you and I hope you enjoy the book.

Janet L. Cumming, Psy.D., President,
Cummings Foundation, and Founder's
Professor, Doctor of Behavioral Health
Program, Arizona State University

# In Appreciation

Both Arizona State University's Doctor of Behavioral Health (DBH) Program and the Cummings Foundation for Behavior Health (CFBH) express their appreciation to Linda Goddard, Executive Assistant at CFBH and Rachel Joles of the staff of the DBH Program, as without their invaluable assistance both the book and program upon which it is based might still be in process.

In recognizing their dedication to appropriate prescribing as well as their understanding of the value of psychotherapy, a special thanks goes to the presenters who participated unselfishly without a rightful and well-earned honorarium so that those funds could be utilized in the publication and greater dissemination of this volume.

# Acknowledgements

The Editors are grateful to Linda Goddard, Executive Assistant, Cummings Foundation for Behavioral Health, for her organizational expertise in the assembly of this book, acting as liaison among the editors, the authors, Arizona State University and Ithaca Press.

A special thanks is owed to Dr. Ronald O'Donnell and his staff at the Nicholas A. Cummings Doctor of Behavioral Health Program, Arizona State University, for the invaluable assistance in organizing the site and conducting the registration and attendance of the Conference upon which this book is based.

# About the Authors
(The Conference Faculty)

**Nicholas A. Cummings, Ph.D., Sc.D.** is a visionary who for half a century not only was able to foresee the future of professional psychology, but helped create it. A former President of the American Psychological Association (APA) as well as its Divisions 12 (Clinical) and 29 (Psychotherapy), he formed 23 national organizations, including the National Academies of Practice, in response to trends. He launched the professional school movement when he founded the four campuses of the California School of Professional Psychology (now Alliant University), and he founded the National Council of Schools of Professional Psychology. After serving as chief of mental health for Kaiser Permanente for 25 years, he then launched American Biodyne, the only psychology-driven national mental health company that grew to 25 million enrollees in 50 states. He has written over 450 journal articles and has published 48 books. He has received scores of honors and awards, including the APA's highest Award for Distinguished Contributions to Practice, as well as the American Psychological Foundation's Gold Medal. In 2008, he collaborated with Arizona State University to found the Doctor of Behavioral Health Program that now bears his name. He is Distinguished Professor at the University of Nevada, Reno.

**David Healy, M.D.** is an Irish psychiatrist and professor of psychiatry at Cardiff University School of Medicine in Wales. He is the Director of the North Wales School of Medicine in Wales. Dr. Healy became the center of controversy concerning the influence of the pharmaceutical industry on medicine and academia with the publication of his book, *Let Them Eat Prozac*. For most of his career, he has held the view that Prozac and SSRIs can lead to suicide and has been highly critical of the amount of ghostwriting in current scientific literature. His views led to what has been termed "The Toronto Affair" that at the core is a debate about academic freedom. His current research interests include cognitive functioning in affective disorders and psychoses as well as circadian rhythms in affective disorders, recovery in psychoses, and physical health of people with mental illness.

**David Antonuccio, Ph.D.** is a professor in the Department of Psychiatry of the Nevada School of Medicine. A Fellow of the American Psychological Association (APA) and an ABPP diplomat in clinical psychology, he is internationally known for his work in depression and smoking cessation. His articles on the comparative effects of psychotherapy and pharmacotherapy have received extensive coverage by the national media and are models of careful scholarship. He was named Outstanding Psychologist by the Nevada State Psychological Association (NSPA) in 1993, received an award of achievement in 1999 from NSPA for his work on depression, was awarded the 2000 McReynolds Foundation Psychological Services Award for "outstanding contributions to clinical science," and received the Association for Psychologists in Academic Health Settings (APAHC) Bud Orgel Award for Distinguished Achievement in Research from the American Psychological Association in 2008. He gratefully acknowledges the participation of Barry Duncan, Psy.D. and his graduate students at the Fielding Institute.

**John Caccavale, Ph.D., M.S.C.P.** is a California-licensed clinical neuropsychologist and the Executive Director of the National Alliance of Professional Psychology Providers (NAPPP). He is a longtime advocate for the advancement of clinical and medical psychology and its inclusion into primary behavioral healthcare. He serves on a number of professional boards, including the American Board of Medical Psychology, the National Institute of Behavioral Health Quality, and the American Board of Behavioral Health Practice. He has published numerous articles and book reviews on a wide array of subjects but, in recent years has confined his writings to the current issues facing the profession in the *Clinical Practitioner*, NAPPP's free monthly newspaper. For his "Failure to Serve" and his controversial, but effective "Truth in Drugs" campaigns, he was presented with the 2011 Cummings PSYCHE Award. Its prestigious roster of the past fourteen recipients, along with it $50,000 prize, render it the highest award in mental health.

**William T. O'Donohue, Ph.D.** is a full professor in the Department of Psychology, University of Nevada, Reno. In the past, he was the Nicholas Cummings Chair of Behavioral Healthcare Delivery at UNR (1999–2007) and president and CEO of CareIntegra (2000–2010). He is an honorary associate professor in the UNR Department of Philosophy, adjunct professor in the Department of Psychiatry, and he maintains a part time private practice in forensic psychology. Outside of Nevada, he is an adjunct professor at the University of Hawaii, Manoa, and the Forest Institute of Professional Psychology in Springfield, Mo. He has authored over 100 articles in refereed journals, over 80 book chapters, and 49 books. He is currently active as a senior fellow of the Cummings Foundation for Behavioral Health.

**Robert B. Whitaker** is a science reporter and writer for the *Albany Times Union* newspaper in New York. He has won numerous awards as a journalist covering medicine and science, including the George Polk Award for Medical Writing and a National Association for Science Writers' Award for best magazine article. In 1998, he co-wrote a series on psychiatric research for the *Boston Globe* that was a finalist for the Pulitzer Prize for Public Service. His book, *Mad in America,* was named by *Discover* magazine as one of the best science books of 2002; the American Library Association named it one of the best history books of that year. His most recent publication, *Anatomy of an Epidemic,* published in 2010, investigates how the use of psychotropic medications has fueled the astounding increases in mentally disabled Americans over the past 50 years.

**Ronald O'Donnell, Ph.D.** is a clinical psychologist and Director of the Nicholas A. Cummings Doctor of Behavioral Health Program at Arizona State University. Prior to his current position, he spent over a decade in health plans as director of care management, disease management, and health coaching programs comprised of behavioral clinicians, physicians, nurses and dieticians designed to improve the outcome of patients with co-morbid medical and behavioral chronic illness. He spent nearly a decade as clinical director for HMO staff model mental health and substance abuse treatment centers closely allied to primary care offices. Early in his career, he treated patients with serious and persistent mental illness in a state hospital and community mental healthcare center settings. O'Donnell has dedicated his career to integrated behavioral care, using outcome management to demonstrate the value-added proposition for behavioral care, and interdisciplinary collaboration.

**Joseph M. Casciani, Ph.D.** is the president of CoHealth. org, a training and education company devoted to integrating health insights, approaches, and principles in the overall health-care of older adults. CoHealth.org's sister companies, Concept Healthcare Psychology Group, Inc. and CoHealth Psychology Services, P.A., hire behavioral health and behavioral medicine practitioners to deliver services to residents in long-term care facilities and also offer extended staff support, training and consultation in these facilities. He has over twenty-five years specializing in the provision of behavioral healthcare with older adults and their families, clinical program development, staff education, and training. He remains one of the nation's most respected authorities on the extensive, integrated care of older adults.

**William E. Pelham, Jr., Ph.D.** is a Distinguished Professor of Psychology at the University of Buffalo and the Director of the Center for Children and Families, an interdisciplinary with faculty and student involvement from the departments of psychology, psychiatry, pediatrics, and pharmacy. His area of interest is attention deficit disorder (ADHD) in children and adolescents. He has studied many facets of ADHD, including the nature of the cognitive deficit, peer relationships, diagnosis, motivation and persistence, family factors, service delivery, and outcomes. He is a Fellow of both the American Psychological Association (APA) and the Association for Psychological Science (APS), and a past president of the Society of Child and Adolescent Clinical Psychology, the International Society for Research in Child and Adolescent Psychopathology, and the Professional Group for Attention Deficit and Related Disorders. He currently serves on the APA's Council of Representatives, as well as the APA Task Force on Medication and Psychosocial Treatments for Children. He founded and directs the biennial Niagara Conference on Evidence Based Treatments for Child and Adolescent Mental Health Problems.

# Table of Contents

Introduction

# Toward the Restoration of Psychotherapy as First Line Treatment

*(Not originally part of the Conference, but added for this publication)*

*William T. O'Donohue, Ph.D.*
*Nicholas A. Cummings, Ph.D., Sc.D.*

I t is the main argument of this book that many patients in the current healthcare system are not receiving the behavioral health treatment that they need (see also Institute of Medicine, 2002). Instead, many patients are receiving interventions that are less effective, less safe, often more costly, and that, perhaps most importantly, have serious and sometimes even lethal side effects (Whittaker, 2010). Among these patients being systematically and routinely mistreated are our nation's children (see Pelham, this volume). Also among these patients are our nation's elderly (see Casciani, this volume). Finally, among these patients being mistreated are our nation's seriously mentally ill (Whittaker, 2010). In other words, often the individuals experiencing the burden of this improper healthcare are our nation's most vulnerable populations. However, no one is immune from this mistreatment, as the depressed college student or the socially anxious carpenter can also be gravely mistreated.

And let us be perfectly clear: the consequences of this mistreatment are not minor. The chapters of this book will make the case that this mistreatment can be deadly or severely debilitating. At a minimum, individuals continue to suffer from their unidentified behavioral health problem instead of receiving the safest, most effective treatment that the healthcare system could, and should, provide. This book is an attempt to call attention to this problematic aspect of our current healthcare system—i.e., to document another dimension of the healthcare crisis (see Cummings & O'Donohue, 2011), as well as to suggest a remedy. Of course, we are not the first to point out this kind of problem, although we think this book is one of the most, if not the most, systematic treatment of the problem and its possible solution. A classic and vitally important document that has received wide attention is the Institute of Medicine's (2002) *Crossing the Quality Chasm.* However, this report focused mainly on the physical healthcare system and relatively neglected safety and quality problems in the behavioral healthcare system. But it is important to note that this report estimated that as many as ninety thousand Americans may die each year due to medical errors.

Moreover, this argument does not imply that this unfortunate state of affairs is caused by evil people or evil corporations. But it also does not imply that financial interest, intellectual blinders, and a problematic lack of concern about quality are wholly irrelevant. We all have a role in this problem and we all must innovate, and due to the suffering caused by the present state of affairs, we must innovate sooner rather than later. The old saying of the 1960s seems relevant here: Are you part of the problem or part of the solution? We do wish to argue that it is urgent that the healthcare received by people suffering from behavioral health problems be dramatically changed and changed dramatically so that hundreds of thousands of individuals receive more effective and safer care. The economics of disruption (Christensen, 2009) postulate that the disrupted modality is most often inadvertently complicit in its own disruption. Psychotherapy, too long mired in the 50-minute hour, has lagged far behind in adopting innovations and efficiency that would have rendered it highly competitive with pharmacotherapy.

It is also important to understand that we are not making the argument that psychotherapy ought to be the first line treatment for a number of behavioral health problems because of parochial interest; e.g., because we are psychotherapists and are biased toward psychotherapy, or because we have emotional or intellectual prejudices against medication or the so called "medical model". It is undeniable that for many health problems medications can be safe, effective and efficient and therefore ought to be the first line of treatment (e.g., antibiotics for bacterial infections, insulin for diabetics, beta blockers for certain coronary conditions; the list could go on and on). However, just because traditional medical treatments are *sometimes* the appropriate treatments does not mean that they are *always* the appropriate treatment. The appropriate treatment must be individually determined by rational criteria for each disorder and each patient. We would suggest a pragmatic meta-criterion ought to be used: what is best for the patient is what ought to be delivered as opposed to what is easiest for the practitioner, or what is in the best financial interests of a business entity.

Unfortunately, what interventions, if any, patients receive for the behavioral health problems currently are not a function of rational and pragmatic factors that ought to be determinative.

Currently, there are a wide variety of factors influencing treatment delivery that include:

- The practitioner's irrational preferences. Practitioners are enamored of a certain psychoreligion (Cummings and O'Donohue, 2008) or have been trained only in one treatment modality. An example of this is a patient who receives psychoanalysis for their PTSD when clearly a review of the outcome literature would indicate that exposure therapy is the treatment of choice (Institute of Medicine, 2006).

- Convenience. Sometimes certain therapies are easier to administer than others (e.g., prescribing a medication vs. faithfully implementing a prolonged course of psychotherapy). Sometimes there is missing expertise in the treatment setting (e.g., a lack of behavioral health expertise in the primary care medical setting; see below). However, convenience should not be as determinative as it appears to be currently.

- Differences in availability and access. Obviously, a therapy cannot be delivered if it is not available (e.g., Dialectical Behavior Therapy may not be available to individuals with Borderline Personality Disorder in many rural areas; or applied behavior analytic interventions may not be available to autistic children of the poor). However, it is never appropriate to hammer a screw just because all one has is a hammer. Too often currently, the healthcare system is not set up to deliver the therapies that patients actually need, as will be discussed more in a later section. The availability of optimal therapy raises key questions about professional training, the design of healthcare systems, and scaling certain key treatment options that will be discussed below.

- A lack of information-rich healthcare environments. Too often healthcare professionals do not have the training and information that clearly specifies what therapies are most effective and safest. Instead, they can receive information that is biased; e.g., from drug representatives, from a distorted, outdated, or incomplete medical literature. Key innovations such as the Patient Centered Medical Homes (see Freeman, 2011, for a description) are based on a foundation of improved information technology systems that provide professionals with comprehensive and accurate information so that they can make better treatment recommendations. In addition, electronic health records in which the patients total care is recorded and evaluated is a key to providing safer more effective therapy (Levin & Hanson, 2011). These are in their infancy in physical medicine and beyond the Veterans Administration system, military treatment facilities and a few large healthcare organizations (e.g., Kaiser Permanente on the West Coast or Geisinger in Pennsylvania); they are virtually nonexistent in behavioral health.

- A lack of a patient who is adequately informed and is actively and effectively self-managing their own health. In healthcare, as in all market transactions, ultimately the buyer needs to beware, or at least be somewhat more pragmatically informed about issues such as safety, effectiveness, and cost. One purpose of this book is to educate consumers. We want patients to be able to better understand the often considerable, but generally unappreciated risks they may encounter with certain options that may become involved in their behavioral healthcare and rationally manage these risks instead of passively relying on the opinions of others. When untoward side effects occur, they should not be reluctant to complain and to report them. We believe strongly that patients ultimately need to make decisions about their own healthcare after careful consideration of an accurate and complete analysis of the risk and benefits of their treatment options.

• An over-concern with cost. This is not to say that cost is irrelevant. We will address this issue in more depth in the next section. Our nation is in a healthcare crisis that is partly comprised of runaway costs, amounting to $1.7 trillion in 2010 and growing at a multiple of the general rate of inflation. We need to deliver cost-effective treatments (Cummings & O'Donohue, 2011). However, the cheapest is not always the best. There is a saying: "There is nothing more expensive than a cheap lawyer". Sometimes—repeat, sometimes—this can be true in healthcare, too. Stimulant medications may be cheaper in the short run for a child who suffers from Attention Deficit Hyperactivity Disorder (ADHD) than a trial of cognitive behavior therapy, but the initially more expensive course of CBT may be cheaper in the long run as it is more effective and also because typically it is administered for a much shorter duration (see Pelham, this volume).

## What Factors Ought to Determine Which Treatment is Delivered?

*Therapies that are safe.* Patients should not experience avoidable harm from their therapies, particularly harm that outweighs the benefits of the therapy, harm that could have been avoided, or harm that could have been predicted, but was not (Institute of Medicine, 2001). Patients ought to be fully informed of the potential harm that may occur from their interventions. This is sometimes done, such as in the speed talking that occurs in television commercials regarding side effects of medications, all the while, a series of attractive actors posing as patients are smiling as if to negate the warnings. Legitimate questions can be raised regarding the extent to which this and other methods, such as the pages of tiny print that follow full-page effusive medication advertisements in magazines, are an effective method of providing this important information. The importance of this factor was immortalized in the Hippocratic Oath: "At least do no harm". The chapters in this book make a strong case that the current, unfortunate behavioral healthcare system is not consistent with the Hippocratic Oath.

The chapters in this book by Robert Whittaker, David Healy, David Antonnucio, and William Pelham make the case that the research evidence indicates that the side effects of many of the most commonly prescribed psychotropics have much more serious side effects for many different patient groups than is commonly known. Sometimes these serious negative effects are experienced when the medications are prescribed as indicated by research protocols, sometimes when these are prescribed off label, sometimes when these are prescribed to other populations (e.g. children or pregnant women) than those examined in previous clinical trials, and sometimes when these are prescribed with other medications due to drug interactions. Sometimes, these negative effects include suicide or death. The crisis deepens when one compiles the number of people on these problematic medications, such as children who are taking a variety of medications, but typically stimulations for their alleged ADD or ADHD; children who are taking a variety of anti-depressants, anxiolytics, and antipsychotics for a variety of diagnosed problems; adults and the elderly who for a variety of reasons, but particularly because of the efficiency of how their livers metabolize medications, are on a variety of psychotropics. The scale of the problem is daunting. It may be even be possible that this harmful treatment affects the majority of Americans at some points in their lives.

This problem is deepened because researchers have paid insufficient attention to including adequate safety measures in their research protocols when measuring therapy outcome. Often in drug studies, there are little to no data on chronic use of these medications, yet many patients are prescribed these medications for years or even decades. There are few to no studies of the safety of multiple drugs or commonly prescribed drug "cocktails". There are few data on the effects on key sub-populations such as pregnant women.

Psychotherapy outcome research also suffers from this problem. Most efficacy and effectiveness research does not have an adequate safety assessment in their set of measures. We know from the 1960s that some psychotherapies can be iatrogenic; e.g., there was some evidence that Gestalt encounter groups caused an increase in suicides. In addition, some psychotherapies have been shown to have negative effects such as instilling false memories of sexual abuse (Lilienfeld, Lynn & Lohr, 2004). We suggest that all outcome research include safety assessments so researchers can more adequately provide data on both sides of the coin, benefit as well as harm. This is especially important in outcome research that compares therapies of different modalities, such as a study of psychotherapy versus medications. This is also vital as there are studies, even though they are too few, as cited in chapters in this book, which indicate that psychotherapy in some key cases is safer than medications. However, clearly more research is needed on this important topic.

One reason why this may be the case is that there seems to be a folk notion that medications, including psychotropic medications, are like "magic bullets"; i.e., that these can simply and solely target the problem and leave all other physiology completely unaffected. Generally, we think that the evidence cited in the following chapters suggests that it is reasonable to conclude that current psychotropic drugs are not magic bullets. It is simply naïve for prescribers or consumers to think that the medication will simply and solely target their problem (e.g., their depression) and have no costs or effects on other physiological functions. Additionally, we often know about this lack of magic bullets based on our everyday experience. The caffeine in a cup of coffee can fortunately "cure" our afternoon drowsiness, but also has the unwanted side effects of jitteriness, stomach upsets, and difficulties sleeping that night. In general, the old adage also applies to behavioral health treatments: there is no free lunch. The consumer needs to assess what the costs of the side effects of his or her treatment are. Providers and information-rich delivery systems need to aid the consumer toward this end.

Therapies that are effective. This dimension has received a lot of attention by researchers and increasing attention by others such as professional organizations (in their providing list of evidence-based treatments or evidence-based practice guidelines; see Fisher & O'Donohue, 2007); managed care organizations that promote evidence-based treatment; and quality assurance companies doing quality audits (such as the National Committee for Quality Assurance or NCQA). For example, the American Psychological Association formed a committee to establish criteria for effective and probably ineffective treatments and publish reports on these (Chambless & Ollendick, 2001). The Institute of Medicine (2006) has recently published a review of the outcome research for Post Traumatic Stress Disorder, in which it finds no psychotropic medications as meeting criteria for effectiveness and only cognitive behavior therapy's exposure treatment as having adequate research support for its effectiveness.

However, the chapters in this book illustrate the complexity of the question of the effectiveness of therapy. Sometimes there are too few data; e.g., the effectiveness of treatments for some of the problems of the elderly are a case in point (see Casciani's chapter, this volume). Sometimes the data are simply inconsistent with the notion that the problem can be effectively treated. For example, there are no outcome data indicating that problems such as Anti-social Personality Disorder or Exhibitionism can be effectively treated. Sometimes the data are equivocal, that some aspects of the problem can be improved, while others remain unimproved. Despite the large amount of attention given to the treatment of Borderline Personality Disorders by Dialectical Behavior Therapy, the data are not consistent with a "cure" but rather improvements in a few aspects of the disorder (i.e., parasuicidal gestures). Sometimes data show effectiveness, but the size of the effect is small. Researchers have attempted to derive additional analysis known as "clinical significance" to make sure statistical significance, that can result from small differences in variables as long as there is a sufficient sample size, is not confused with a practical clinical effect. Sometimes the data are conflicting, such as when one study shows a treatment effect, while another shows no effect. These cases are rendered even more difficult to interpret because the quality of the research design varies across studies. How does one interpret a positive treatment effect from a smaller sample with less clear inclusion criteria with a null finding from a study with a larger sample and tighter inclusion criteria?

However, as the chapters in the book illustrate, the story is also more complex and interesting. Because vested interests are involved in the production of a body of outcome literature, this literature is messier and more difficult to interpret than many assume it is. For example, there is the "file drawer" problem. If someone is interested in proving a therapy is effective (say a drug company is interested in showing positive results from one of its drugs), but the observed results of the outcome study indicate a null finding, the study can simply be not submitted for publication. Rather, it is functionally placed in a drawer never to see the light of day. Several chapters in this volume illustrate the "dirty little tricks" that can be played in producing the body of outcome literature, particularly for antidepressant medications. Unfortunately, it seems reasonable to conclude that the phrase "buyer beware" also applies to consumers of outcome information.

The final point to be made in effectiveness has to do with the distinction between efficacy and effectiveness research. Efficacy research is an investigation of the outcomes of an intervention in rather ideal laboratory conditions, such as patients who have no comorbid problems and that clearly meet DSM-IVTR criteria for the disorder. Further, these therapies are delivered by expert therapists often with deep expertise in the therapy as well as loyalty toward them. They are often delivered at no cost and even with extraordinary measures, such as fidelity checks, patients being paid for participation, patients given reminders to increase compliance, and a number of other extraordinary features. These features are generally balanced, or perhaps even weighted, toward increasing the probability that the therapy will be shown to be effective. Effectiveness research per se, on the other hand, is designed to evaluate the outcomes of the therapy in more "real world" settings. Patients can have comorbid conditions, therapists who are not the originators of the therapy, but average practitioners participate, and patients most often pay for their therapy and are given few special perks, such as free transportation. It is important that both kinds of studies be conducted to be able to more accurately assess the effectiveness of a therapy as it would be delivered to actual patients. Knowing only outcome data derived from efficacy studies raises serious questions about the generalizability of these results.

Effectiveness studies also begin to raise the question of scalability of an intervention strategy. These are related to key questions about access as well as cost and thus are vitally important. If a therapy is effective the next question becomes how do we disseminate it to all the people who need it? How many therapists need to be trained to deliver this therapy faithfully? Is this therapy difficult to learn? To what extent do therapists over time drift away from faithful implementation? What is the cost of this training and are therapists available and interested in learning it? The first author has noted that in the introduction of their dissertations, students typically briefly talk about the magnitude of the problem (e.g., "20 million Americans affected"), trends in this (e.g., "and increasing at some dramatic rate"), and the problem's tremendous cost (e.g., "costing an estimated $17 billion in treatment and lost productivity"). After this, they conduct outcome studies of some interventions, and when they get positive results they seem perfectly happy and content. However, all the dots have not been connected. When asked, even assuming further positive studies of the efficacy and effectiveness of this novel intervention, how do they scale it to the millions of suffering individuals they described in their introduction, they are stumped. They usually have not even considered this important problem and have no answer. Scalability is admittedly a very tough issue for psychotherapy. One advantage of medications over psychotherapy is that they have many fewer problems with scalability as the drug company simply produces more pills and primary care doctors prescribe these. Producing skilled therapists who can faithfully implement a therapy system is a much more difficult task.

*Therapies that are efficient.* Therapies should not only be safe and effective they need to be efficient too. Efficiency allows the economic dimension to enter in treatment decisions (Cummings, 2007). Efficiency also requires an analysis of the speed of effects. Our healthcare system simply cannot afford inefficient treatment, because of the unnecessary human suffering and because of the tremendous financial burden. It is interesting that there is a program of research trying to show for example, hundreds of sessions of psychoanalysis have the equivalent effectiveness to about 20 sessions of CBT for problems like anxiety and depression. If one looks only at effectiveness these two therapies appear to be equivalent; however, if one also looks at efficiency then clearly CBT ought to be the preferred treatment.

Clay Christensen (2009) who is probably the most influential thinker in President Obama's attempts at healthcare reform has indicated that given the epidemiological findings about the frequency of health problems in the American population, we cannot reform healthcare simply by disseminating traditional treatments to more individuals. Rather, Christensen argues that we must redesign the current healthcare system to allow patients access to a variety of more efficient alternatives. For example, seeing a nurse practitioner for a probable case of strep throat is more efficient than seeing a pediatrician. In behavioral health, it is more efficient to be seen in group therapy for cases of mild depression than to be seen individually (Cummings, 2008). Also, Cummings in his statement of the patient bill of rights has said that patients and practitioners need to be committed to the following principle: "The patient is entitled to relief from pain, anxiety, and depression in the shortest time possible and with the least intrusive intervention." Thus, patients and other stakeholders also need to have and to consider data regarding the interventions speed and cost when considering what therapies ought to be delivered.

*Therapies need to be designed and implemented with a consideration of patient preferences.* We agree with the notion, often implied if not stated in subsequent chapters in this book, that the patient ought to be empowered to make their healthcare decisions. It is paternalistic to assume that patients will be passive and simply follow the "doctor's orders". After all, it is the patient who has to live (hopefully) with the outcomes of these healthcare decisions. Thus, we believe that in an improved healthcare system significant efforts are made to assure that patients (or their guardians) are given key information on treatment options as well as accurate information on safety, effectiveness, the speed of effects, cost, availability, and other key dimensions. It is arguable that our current ethical codes imply that this ought to happen as part of the informed consent process. However, in practice this is often neglected or done in an inadequate manner. Some have lamented that currently Americans have more access to information about the quality of books and movies (through such sources as amazon. com and Netflix.com; rottentomatoes.com) than they do regarding their healthcare options. This is quite problematic.

*Therapies that increase the likelihood that the patient will become an active participant in the management of their health.* Patients ultimately need to be empowered with the information and skills to manage their own health. Patients make numerous micro-decisions each day regarding their health: should they exercise today? Should they drink the fourth cocktail? Should they eat another 500 calories? Should they take the third dose of their medication as prescribed? Healthcare professionals cannot simply follow every American around helping them to make healthy choices. Ultimately, each person must make these and it can be the job of healthcare professionals to instill skills so that they increasingly do so. Many critics of the present day medical system complain that it is a "sickness care system" rather than a "healthcare system" as it does little to increase the probability of current or future health. Rather it waits until sickness occurs and then becomes activated by treating this sickness. Critics point out that an absence of sickness does not mean a presence of health. The substance of the criticism is rather straightforward: it may be cheaper to prevent a problem than to manage or cure it; and it is certainly in the person's best interest to completely avoid sickness rather than experience some degree of it that is then cured.

However, in enacting this reform the devil is in the details. It is not clear that we currently have the technology to prevent behavioral health problems. Certainly more research is needed in safe, effective and efficient prevention methods. For example, there are some data (although some aspects are increasingly controversial) that physical checkups are useful in early detection or prevention of certain physical health problems. However, we don't have the equivalent data or process in behavioral health. What would an annual behavioral health check-up look like? Would its cost be justified by the benefits it produces?

*Therapies need to prioritize the patients' problems and not miss the most severe threats to patients' functioning and wellbeing.* This is the healthcare equivalent of rearranging the deck chairs on the *Titanic*. It makes no sense in a medical environment to treat a slightly infected hang nail when an artery has been severed in another part of the body and the patient is bleeding to death. Similarly it makes no sense to treat a patient's existential dilemma when the patient is a severe alcoholic. As another example, it is also unreasonable to only treat a patients' marital dissatisfaction when they are severely obese and their diabetes is not being managed properly. The entire behavioral health of a patient needs to be thoroughly and comprehensively assessed and although DSM conditions need to be identified; the patients behavioral health problems such as lifestyle problems (smoking included), treatment compliance problems, and other behavioral health problems (e.g., chronic pain) need to be identified and properly prioritized in a holistic and properly prioritized treatment plan.

*Therapies need to be delivered in a timely manner.* Currently there is a shortage of psychiatrists and in some locales, waits for an appointment can be in the range of 3–6 months. This is not timely behavioral treatment. One reason why the primary care medical clinic is the *de facto* mental health system in our country is that treatment has the potential to be much timelier. Primary care clinics are better distributed geographically and waits for appointments are usually much less than in specialty care. However, sometimes primary care clinics also have inordinate waiting time, particularly inordinate when someone is in pain. We need to figure out how to deliver safe, effective, efficient therapy that patients prefer, in a timely manner.

*Therapies that the therapist is competent to provide.* Unfortunately, it is unreasonable for consumers to assume that just because a therapy is evidence-based and the professional has a behavioral health degree, that the professional is competent to provide that therapy. Too few therapists are trained in evidence-based treatments (Chambless & Ollendick, 2001; Fisher & O'Donohue, 2007). Some therapists knowing what is "hot" can simply claim that they know this treatment and give a "college try" and attempt to implement what is their (often incomplete or mistaken) understanding of the therapy. Or even more problematically use "bait and switch" techniques in which they simply relabel what they usually provide as the evidence-based therapy. There are no clear quality indicators of professional competence in delivering key evidence-based therapies.

Gwande (2009) has made the argument that a key in healthcare quality is the number of times the healthcare professional has administered the treatment. He points out that all new skills involve a learning curve; and that the problem in healthcare is real patients are components of each stage of the learning curve. In his analysis, one of the most important questions a potential patient needs to assess is the number of times the practitioner has delivered the intervention. Answers that allay concerns are in the several hundreds if not thousands. This implies that quality is found in specialization and that general practitioners—what many therapists are in our field—can have a particularly difficult time in achieving excellence and perhaps even competence. Thus another issue in our field is how do we measure practitioner competence? How do we help practitioners achieve competence and excellence? Is part of the answer to this question inevitably that of specialization?

## Integrated Care

Currently, the subsequent chapters of this book argue many patients receive sub-optimal care because the healthcare system is not designed to give them better care. There are many design flaws in the current healthcare system, e.g., a lack of quality information systems supporting electronic health records, but a key design flaw is the lack of quality behavioral health in medical settings (see Cummings & O'Donohue, 2011). When behavioral health is properly coordinated with medical care, then the delivery system can be said to be integrated.

Integrated care has the potential of restoring behavioral health to the first line treatment of many behavioral health disorders because it includes a behavioral health specialist in the medical team to more properly identify behavioral health pathways of the medical presentation (O'Donohue, et al, 2006). In addition, it provides the patient with treatment options. In a fractionated care system, the physician can either refer the patient to an external mental health profession or give the patient psychotropic medications. Many of the subsequent chapters contained in this book tell the story of the many problems with this unnecessarily restricted choice. The data on patients following through with these external referrals are dismal as only about 25% do (Cummings, 2008). In addition, the efficacy and safety of these psychotropic medications is quite problematic.

Redesigning healthcare to include behavioral health so that it is integrated in medical settings is critical as the primary care medical setting is the de facto mental healthcare system in the United States. Most psychotropic medications are prescribed by primary care physicians and not by psychiatrists. Patients like one-stop shopping and they trust their primary care physician (Cummings, O'Donohue et al, 2005). In addition, primary care clinics are more ubiquitous and thus allow more patients access to care.

Thus, integrated care settings can better achieve the criteria that we listed above for higher quality treatment:

- Integrated healthcare can provide safer care by allowing patients to try courses of safer treatment such as psychotherapy.
- Integrated settings can provide more effective care by providing a fuller array of treatment options; e.g., exposure therapy for PTSD instead of an ineffective anxiolytic.
- Integrated care can provide more efficient therapy, by more accurately identifying what the patient's actual problems are through comprehensive assessments of patients' physical problems and behavioral health problems. In this manner, for example, anxious patients can be given effective treatments for their anxiety instead of being sent to cardiologists with their concerns about their episodes of increased heart rates.
- Integrated care can provide delivery systems in which patients' preferences are better incorporated by providing patients with more treatment options. Instead of only being told of psychotropic medication options, the patient can now be educated regarding legitimate psychotherapy options.

- Integrated care can aid the patients in self-managing their health by both more comprehensively identifying pathways to improved health (e.g., stop smoking, increased exercise, better diet), but also by using behavioral interventions to directly improve skills in disease management and healthcare.

- Integrated healthcare settings can help properly prioritize a patient's healthcare problems by comprehensively looking at both physical and behavioral health problems. When there is a collocated behavioral health professional in the primary care setting their mental health and behavioral health problems can be better identified.

- Integrated care can provide timelier care because a behavioral health professional can be immediately called into the exam room and instantly begin the assessment and treatment of the patient's behavioral health issues. Instead of waiting for an external referral to be accepted, the patient is seen, and information flows back to the physician, and the team can address the behavioral health concerns in matters of minutes.

- Integrated care can provide therapy that the therapist is competent to deliver. Training curricula have been developed and implemented (see O'Donnell, this volume). Clinicians need to be monitored to make sure they have the full range of skills and are delivering high quality interventions within the primary care treatment model. However, it is also important to note that the team approach allows more light to be shown on what treatments are being delivered.

Thus, we argue that integrated care is the key to restoring psychotherapy to its proper place as a first line treatment. Although there are many useful introductions to integrated care

(O'Donohue, et al, 2006; Robinson & Reiter, 2006), many people still misunderstand integrated care. In the next section, we will briefly review some of the major myths regarding integrated care in order allay the major misunderstandings about it.

## The Top Myths about Integrated Care

*Myth 1: Integrated care is simply placing mental health professionals in a medical setting and allowing these practitioners to practice as usual.*
This is probably the most frequently mistaken idea. This is not integrated care. This service delivery model might have a few advantages, but by and large, this is a recipe for a lot of frustration and disappointment. Only integrated care done properly will deliver the outcomes stakeholders generally want from integration. These are improved patient care, physician satisfaction, efficiency, patient satisfaction, and medical cost reduction. Integrated care needs to be designed and delivered quite differently from simply allowing a specialty mental health practitioner to practice as they do in specialty settings. In integrated behavioral health, providers need to acquire special skills to work in an integrated setting:

- The integrated behavioral health providers need to be medically-oriented. They need to be medically literate and oriented to medical presentations such as treatment non-adherence, pain management, chronic disease management, lifestyle change. These clinicians cannot just be simply oriented to DSM diagnostic problems as they are in a specialty mental health practice.
- When behavioral health providers assess and treat mental health problems they need to do this in the same ecological style as the primary care medical set-

ting: fast-paced, action-oriented, and driven toward population management.

- Behavioral health providers will rarely use the 50-minute hour. Rather patients should be scheduled similarly to the fast pace of primary care practice, such as in 15 minute blocks.
- Integrated care clinicians often use a consultation liaison model to support the physician in a more comprehensive assessment and treatment of the patient, instead of a specialty care treatment model. The patient remains the physician's patient and the integrated care practitioner is part of the healthcare team.
- The medical team can interrupt the behavioral health provider and expect to get answers to their referral questions from the behavioral health provider in less than an hour.
- Behavioral health providers need to practice as part of a team, as the most important customer of the integrated care professional is the medical team.
- The primary care behavioral health treatment provider needs to use evidence-based protocols, for as previously noted, not all mental health professionals do. Integrated care will only be as good as the assessments and interventions the clinician uses. If problematic assessments are transported into an integrated care setting, they will fail. The interventions the integrated care practitioner provides need to meet all the criteria delineated in the previous section; i.e., these interventions need to be safe, effective, efficient, oriented toward self-management, etc.
- They need to conduct their services with feedback regarding outcomes and quality improvement processes (see O'Donohue, Ammirati, & Lilienfeld, 2011). We

recommend constant feedback to assure that there is no drift toward problematic practices and to measure the degree to which each clinician is achieving the goals of integrated care.

There are other differences, but this ought to give the reader a flavor that integrated care is quite a different healthcare delivery paradigm. It can be successfully implemented, but the devil is in the details. With proper hiring, training, and supervision, it can perform in a manner that produces the desired outcomes (see James and O'Donohue, 2008).

*Myth 2: Integrated care is a new delivery model and has not been shown to produce medical savings.*

This is false. Nicholas Cummings, Ph.D., former APA President, designed integrated care clinics for Kaiser Permanente in the 1960s. In addition, a number of large treatment systems have integrated care over the past few decades, such as the U.S. Air Force, V.A. system, Kaiser Permanente, Group Health, etc. In the past decade, the interest in integrated care has exploded. It has gone from a relatively novel concept, to one that is much more understood and accepted. There are over two dozen studies showing significant savings. These data are summarized in Cummings, O'Donohue & Ferguson (2002), *The Impact of Medical Cost Offset on Practice and Research: Making It Work for You.*

*Myth 3: Integrated behavioral health and disease management are the same things. If an organization is doing one; it does not have to do the other.*

This is incorrect. Contemporary disease management is valuable, as it often provides information and support to patients struggling with chronic diseases such as diabetes, asthma, and depression. However, it is also often "treatment-lite". It uses only the lowest steps in a stepped care model (see next section) and can improve a lot of the patient problems amenable to interventions using educational and support pathways. However, there are other pathways to high medical utilization for individuals suffering from chronic diseases and often require a more "high touch", more intensive assessment and treatment. Examples are serious co-morbidities such as substance abuse, and for undiagnosed behavioral health problems such as Personality Disorders. Integrated care fills this gap in disease management programs by providing the clinical services these patients need in the setting they prefer, meaning the primary care medical setting. Integrated care is not parachuting one or two disease management protocols into a medical service delivery system.

*Myth 4: If an organization integrates care there is no need for specialty behavioral health anymore.*

Just as if a primary care physician may manage some low level cardiac problems (e.g., angina and high blood pressure) without involving a cardiologist, but for more acute or more serious problems will refer to a cardiologist, integrated behavioral health operates the same manner. Specialty care behavior health is still needed as most, but not all, chronic behavioral health problems such as bipolar, schizophrenic, autistic, conduct disordered, and suicidal patients. These patients are still most often best handled in specialty behavioral health. The co-located integrated care specialist will help triage and manage the referral of these patients to specialty behavioral health.

*Myth 5: Integrated care will not produce medical cost offset.*

The research literature is clear. If the integrated care delivery system is designed and implemented correctly, integrated care produces reductions in total healthcare costs. These reductions can be significant. The literature indicates the range is around

20–40%, depending upon populations served, such as outreached high utilizers vs. physician referred primary care patients (Cummings, O'Donohue & Ferguson, 2002). However, these savings are in no way automatic. They only can be produced with the right clinicians, trained and monitored in the right manner, and using the right clinical models. High quality, evidenced-based targeted medically-oriented treatments are critical.

*Myth 6: Financial models for integrated care are not developed.*

It is true that this is a relatively novel paradigm. However, there are at least three ways this model can be financed: (a) Through the use of the mental health benefit. Many patients, although certainly not all, that require treatment in an integrated care setting have legitimate DSM diagnoses. (b) Through agreements (risk arrangements can vary) that invest in establishing integrated care so that medical costs reductions can be achieved and these savings shared. (c) Through the use of the ICD behavioral health consultation codes:

# The Health and Behavior Assessment and Intervention Codes

96150 – the initial assessment of the patient to determine the biological, psychological, and social factors affecting the patient's physical health and any treatment problems.

96151 – a re-assessment of the patient to evaluate the patient's condition and determine the need for further treatment. A re-assessment may be performed by a clinician other than the one who conducted the patient's initial assessment.

96152 – the intervention service provided to an individual to modify the psychological, behavioral, cognitive, and social factors affecting the patient's physical health and wellbeing. Examples include increasing the patient's awareness about his or her disease and using cognitive and behavioral approaches to initiate physician prescribed diet and exercise regimens.

96153 – the intervention service provided to a group. An example is a smoking cessation program that includes educational information, cognitive-behavioral treatment and social support. Group sessions typically last for 90 minutes and involve 8 to 10 patients.

96154 – the intervention service provided to a family with the patient present. For example, a psychologist could use relaxation techniques with both a diabetic child and his or her parents to reduce the child's fear of receiving injections and the parents' tension when administering the injections.

96155 – the intervention service provided to a family without the patient present. An example would be working with parents and siblings to shape the diabetic child's behavior, such as praising successful diabetes management behaviors and ignoring disruptive tactics.

Until now, almost all intervention codes used by psychologists involved psychotherapy and required a mental health diagnosis, such as under the DSM-IV. In contrast, health and behavior assessment and intervention services focus on patients whose primary diagnosis is physical in nature. Use of the codes will enable reimbursement for the delivery of psychological services for an individual whose problem is a physical illness and does not have a mental health diagnosis. Increasingly, insurers are reimbursing behavioral health professionals for these codes in order to achieve the benefits of integrated care.

**Myth 7: Integrated care is just more managed care and will suffer all of the same problems.**
Integrated care is different because it is a supply side solution to rising medical costs, not a demand side solution. That is, integrated care attempts to give the patient *more* care (behavioral care that they need, but are not getting) so that in the future, they are healthier and need *less* care. This should make integrated care more palatable to many stakeholders. Integrated care is necessary as many patients need behavioral care for problems such as:

- Help with treatment compliance
- Help with acute or chronic pain management
- Intense disease management
- Help with depression and anxiety
- Help with lifestyle change (diet, exercise, smoking)
- Help with general stress, including stress from having a medical problem
- Help with caregiving (children, elderly patients)
- Case management

Patients who are not treated in integrated care settings typically do not get these from their physical medicine visits. If any of these are a pathway causing the visit, more and more physical medicine can be prescribed to these individuals, resulting in huge costs, but not much benefit. Integrated care can provide these services resulting in a healthier lower-utilizing patient.

# Stepped Care

Evidence-based stepped care has great potential to also provide a higher quality delivery system and to restore psychotherapy to a first line intervention. A stepped care delivery system is one in which treatment options are organized in a hierarchy of intensity that usually also correlates with cost. Patients then can be triaged based on some relevant criteria, such as severity, cost or choice, to a certain step. It is also generally recognized that is acceptable to "fail upwards," i.e., that a certain step can be tried and if the problem is refractory at this step, then a more intense step can be attempted next.

An example might be useful of evidence-based stepped care. For Major Depressive Episode the steps might be:

1. Watchful waiting for mild cases that are perhaps trending toward improvement, with no suicidal ideation or history, with a patient who is willing to wait a few weeks to see if there is improvement. But the patient can call in immediately for other steps if the condition worsens.

2. Psycho-education materials such as pamphlets that give information about depression and what might be done (e.g., behavioral activation, exercise, gaining increased social support).

3. Bibliotherapy. Books such as David Burn's (1999) excellent *Feeling Good* that have outcome research (Scogin, Hamblin, & Beutler, 1987; Jamison & Scogin 1995; Ackerson et al 1998) that are accessible quickly and cheaply that essentially are cognitive behavioral interventions put in a self-help format.

4. E-health. There are websites such as moodgym.com that have more involved therapies that may be inexpensive or even free, and that also instantiate cognitive behavioral treatments.

5. Group therapy. Group therapies are more efficient than individual therapy and often have similar outcome and patient satisfaction.

6. Individual outpatient therapy. This is of course the modal form of intervention in specialty mental health and has its place in stepped care. Stepped care approaches though assume that it is over used given that the delivery system is not properly structured to demonstrate alternatives

7. Medication is one of the most utilized interventions because most depression is treated in the primary care medical setting (Katon et al, 1997). Part of the reform has to be to design evidence-based stepped care systems for primary care so that primary care physicians can give alternatives to their patients.

8. Inpatient therapy is expensive and costly in terms of altering the patient's life, but sometimes it is necessary due to severity of the problem, especially given suicidal behavior.

More research is needed regarding triage. Is there some sort of patient matching that would be predictive of best outcomes? Currently, we believe that professionals should show patients all these options and engage in conjoint decision making to decide upon an initial step. Then patient progress should be closely monitored (by patient or professional) to decide whether another step should be considered. At times, multiple steps can be tried together, such as bibliotherapy plus medication as just one example.

We believe it is evident how stepped care, particularly when practiced in an integrated care setting, can better accomplish the quality criteria we listed earlier in this chapter. It can provide therapies that are safer, timelier, more effective, more efficient, and that more accurately prioritize patient problems, with more patient choice, and that therapists are actually competent to provide. However, more research is clearly needed to evaluate the outcomes of these integrated care, stepped care systems.

# References

Burns, D. (1999). *Feeling good: The new mood therapy*. New York: Harper.

Chambless, D. & Ollendick, T.H. (2001). Empirically supported psychological interventions: Controversies and evidence. *Annual Review of Psychology*. 685-716.

Christensen, C.M., with Grossman, J.H. & Hwang, J. (2009). *The innovator's prescription: A disruptive solution for healthcare*. New York: McGraw Hill.

Cummings, N.A. (2007). Treatment and assessment taken place in an economic context: Always. In S. Lilienfeld & W. O'Donohue (Eds). *The great ideas of clinical in clinical science.* New York: Routledge.

Cummings, N.A. & O'Donohue, W. (2008). *Eleven blunders that cripple psychotherapy: A remedial unblundering*. New York: Routledge.

Cummings, N.A. O'Donohue, W. & Ferguson. K. (Eds.) (2002). *The impact of medical cost offset on practice and research: Making it work for you*. Reno, NV: Context Press.

Cummings, N.A. & O'Donohue, W. (Eds.) (2011). *Understanding the behavioral healthcare crisis: The promise of integrated care and diagnostic reform*. New York: Routledge.

Fisher, J.E., & O'Donohue. W. (Eds.) (2006*). Practitioner's guide to evidence based treatments*. New York: Springer.

Freeman, D. (2011). The behavioral health medical home. In N.A. Cummings & W. O'Donohue (Eds.). *Understanding the behavioral healthcare crisis: The promise of integrated care and diagnostic reform*. New York: Routledge.

Gwanda, A. (2003). *Complications: A surgeon's notes on an imperfect science*. New York: Picador.

Institute of Medicine (2001). *Crossing the quality chasm: A new healthcare system for the 21st century*. Washington, D.C: The National Academies Press.

Institute of Medicine. (2006). *PTSD: Diagnosis and treatment*. Washington: D.C. The National Academies Press.

James L. & O'Donohue, W. (Eds.) (2008). *The primary care toolbox*. New York: Springer.

Jamison, C., & Scogin, F. (1995). The outcome of cognitive bibliotherapy with depressed adults. *Journal of Consulting and Clinical Psychology*, 63(4), 644-650.

Katon, W., Korff, M. V., Lin, E., Unützer, J., Simon, G., Ludman, E., et al. (1997). Population-based care of depression: Effective disease management strategies to decrease prevalence. *General Hospital Psychiatry*, *19*(3), 169-178.

Levin, B.L. & Hanson, A. (2011). Mental health informatics. In N.A. Cummings & W._O'Donohue (Eds.) *Understanding the behavioral healthcare crisis: The promise of integrated care and diagnostic reform*. New York: Routledge

Lilienfeld, S, Lynn, S.J. & Lohr, J. (Eds.) (2004). *Science and pseudoscience in clinical psychology*. New York: Guilford.

O'Donohue, W., Cummings, N.A., Cucciarre, M., Runyan, C., & Cummings, J. (2006). *Integrated behavioral healthcare: A guide to effective intervention*. New York: Prometheus.

O'Donohue, W., Ammirati, R., & Lilienfeld, S. (2011). The quality improvement agenda in behavioral healthcare reform. In. N.A. Cummings & W. O'Donohue (Eds). *Understanding the behavioral healthcare crisis: The promise of_integrated care and diagnostic reform.* New York: Routledge

Robinson, P. & Reiter, J. (2006). *Behavioral health consultation in primary care*. New York: Springer.

Scogin, F., Hamblin, D., & Beutler, L. (1987). Bibliotherapy for depressed older adults: A self-help alternative. *The Gerontologist*, 27(3), 383-387.

Whittaker, R. (2010). *The anatomy of an epidemic*. New York: Crown.

Chapter 1

# Psychotherapy: How It Was and How It Was Disrupted.

*Is Another Disruption Imminent that Will Restore Psychotherapy as the First Line Intervention in Behavioral Care?*

*Nicholas A. Cummings, Ph.D., Sc.D.*

The economics of disruption, or how the new replaces the old, has been a subject of interest for some time, but it is only recently that economist Clayton Christensen (2009) and his medical colleagues have addressed specifically the manner in which this occurs in healthcare. By definition, when economic disruption occurs, a successful, often long established industry, product, or delivery system is abruptly replaced by a newer, more advanced, and more desirable invention, design, or concept. This change is most often accompanied by a painful transition for the displaced in the loss of jobs, income, and recognition. The classic example cited in history is that of the telegraph system that spanned the continent and brought communication down to a matter of minutes instead of weeks. Then came the invention of the telephone that made possible actual voice conversation instead of the dot-dash of the Morse Code. The telegraph lines had spanned the nation and could easily have been converted to accommodate the telephone, but the telegraph company was bloated with success and rejected the idea. We all know the outcome: by disruption, the telephone company rapidly replaced the telegraph. Illustrations of economic disruption abound with such innovations as air travel, copying machines, the personal computer, television, and on and on.

Before the twentieth century, medicine was largely intuitive; that is, physicians diagnosed by symptoms and without the verification of objective tests or devices that diagnosed actual diseases. The absence of objective verification led to early diagnoses such as "bad blood" for which leeches were the only treatment. And since it was the only treatment available, death of the patient was always attributed to the "bad blood" and not the loss of blood through leeching. From the initial stethoscope and similar primitive devices, medicine now has at its disposal a vast array of objective devices from ever-increasingly sophisticated laboratory tests to hand-held imaging. Thus, in the last century *intuitive* medicine was replaced by *objective* medicine, and the previous too often arbitrary syndromes were replaced by actual diseases.

The last branch of medicine that remains shamefully intuitive is psychiatry, shamefully because of its attempts to demonstrate pseudo-objectivity. The Diagnostic and Statistical Manuals (DSMs) are composed of arbitrary groupings of symptoms that are assigned medical sounding syndrome names, and are periodically shuffled, increased, and renamed, while none have any objectively determined efficacy to actual diseases.

Originally psychiatry was primarily a psychotherapy profession like psychology, but differed in that it could also prescribe and hospitalize. As health insurance began to reimburse patients for psychotherapy costs, it became imperative to arrive at a standard nomenclature that was recognizable to all practitioners, and one the health insurance industry could use to pay for care. This objective was laudable, and the DSM-I in the 1950s met that purpose. How the successive DSMs became more and more for-every-syndrome-there-is-a-medication has been termed "the medicalization of psychiatry" that began in the 1970s, but took hold in the decades following 1980, to the extent that today, psychotherapy has been largely displaced by psychotropic medications. How and why this occurred will be described, but first it would be well to see how it once was and how this was disrupted.

## The Golden Age of Psychotherapy

It comes as a surprise to today's practitioners when they learn that the Golden Age of Psychotherapy was the decade of the 1950s. In spite of there being no licensure or insurance reimbursement, there are a number of reasons why this was so, that have never been published or otherwise disseminated. Having gone into private practice in 1948, I lived that era that saw the birth and development of non-medical psychotherapy. In essence, then, this chapter is in part the personal journal of one who lived the birth and current near demise of our profession as a flourishing practice. Additionally, I was privileged to serve on President Kennedy's mental health task force, President Carter's Mental Health Commission and served as an adviser to Senator Edward (Ted) Kennedy's Senate Subcommittee on Health, and Senator Russell Long's Senate Finance Committee all in the crucial years in which the importance of mental health was being established. Further, I served as American Psychological Association (APA) president in 1979 when the medicalization of psychiatry was taking hold and replacing psychotherapy with medications, as well as serving on the APA Council of Representatives and the APA Board of Directors the years preceding. If that were not enough, I was also the psychologist adviser to the Association for the Advancement of

Psychiatry (AAP) and the only psychologist on the blue-ribbon American Psychiatric Association's (ApA) committee chaired by Byrum Karasu that was formulating the ApA's official manual listing and describing the "approved" psychotherapies.

Before World War II, there were less than 200 psychologists in private practice scattered throughout the United States. Most were women treating children, and all but four were master's level practitioners. Two of these four doctoral psychologists were Nancy Bailey and Florence Mateer, both of whom became my early mentors and subsequently my colleagues and friends. The chief psychiatrist for the military in WW II was (Brigadier General) William "Will" Menninger, brother of Karl, and co-founder of the famed Menninger Clinic in Topeka, Kansas. (The unbelievable demise in the late 1980s of mental health's most famous private institution is a story in itself of how it became a victim of medicalization). Menninger advanced psychiatry and psychology seemingly overnight as he (a) expanded medicine and surgery departments to include departments of psychiatry in every facility for the first time, (b) established the School of Military Neuropsychiatry on Long Island, New York, and brought the finest practitioners of the time there as faculty, and (c) trained master's level psychologists to serve as early interventionists with what we now call PTSD, or post-traumatic stress syndrome, right on the front lines.

## Psychology Invades America

Post WW II American society was so captivated by the advances in psychotherapy made in the military that psychotherapy became the favorite subject of motion pictures, magazines, novels and almost daily news items. The Veterans Administration (V.A.) created programs in clinical psychology and positions in doctoral level psychology, and the newly established National Institute of Mental Health (NIMH) funded scores of clinical psychology programs in universities in an effort to meet the burgeoning demand. I was one of those returning veterans who became interested in psychology through my war experiences, and when I went back to school it was in clinical psychology, not to medical school as I had completed premedical studies before entering the army. Studying under the G.I. Bill, I was one of the hordes of returning veterans who established the profession of clinical psychology, along with non-medical psychotherapy.

It was a remarkable era. There was no problem in establishing an independent practice as there was such a tremendous demand in the face of a shortage of practitioners. Fees for psychiatrists were fifteen dollars for a fifty minute hour and ten dollars for the emerging practice of psychology, a level at that time suitable to both patient and doctor as insurance was non-existent. The media loved us, and almost weekly I was interviewed for an article or asked to do a five minute radio tape that would be broadcast over and over again. Of course there was no TV at the time, but popular magazines regularly featured psychology. One popular women's magazine held a poll every year to determine who their readers thought would make the best husband, and psychologist came in number one for eleven straight years. We were society's new heroes.

Social workers did not begin to enter private practice until decades later; and marriage and family therapists (MFTs) and counselors did not exist. There was an even greater shortage of psychiatrists, and our only competition was the occasional quack that managed to get listed in the Yellow Pages of the phonebook, but was quickly marginalized. Psychology had it all: prestige, practice, autonomy. And since there was no licensure, there was not even a bureaucracy, reasonable or unreasonable, to intrude or bother us. Since APA was not involved, practicing psychologists banded together and formed our own referral systems and ethical practice standards. These informal groups later became our local and state associations. This was truly our Golden Era.

Later, as competition increased, with the inevitable conflict arising between psychiatry and psychology, it became imperative that we establish psychology licensure, eligibility for government positions, and insurance reimbursement. There ensued several decades of struggle to obtain these, as we had to fight not only the opposition of the ApA, but also the indifference and even obstruction of our own APA. This fight was led by the Dirty Dozen, who were actually 14 valiant psychologist activists who had to resort to guerilla tactics over two decades, and is beyond the scope of this chapter. It is extensively chronicled in the *Practice of Psychology: The Battle for Professionalism* (Wright & Cummings, 2001). Originally the term Dirty Dozen was intended to be pejorative, pointing to the aggressiveness of the struggle, but the group of 14 seized upon the name calling as a badge of honor. Their successes did, indeed, elevate the name as the surviving members of the Dirty Dozen were honored in a special ceremony by the APA in the late 1990s. It was there that we were awarded the distinction of having valiantly established the modern concept of professional psychology. Along with this, and inadvertently perhaps, the Dirty Dozen had established the practice of non-medical psychotherapy for the professions of social work and counseling that followed.

## How We Practiced

The early professional psychologists pretty much designed practices patterned after those established by Sigmund Freud in Vienna. There was no receptionist, and when a prospective patient called to make an appointment they were connected to an answering machine, the predecessor of today's voicemail. When free, the psychologist called the patient back and a first appointment was scheduled. The patient was instructed to come to the office and take a seat in the waiting room, and he/she would be called exactly at the appointment hour. Since this was a solitary practice with no receptionist, there would be no one else in the waiting room. The previous patient left through an exit that insured the departing and arriving patients would not see each other. The arriving patient was ushered through a double door, one opening inward and the other outward, and the insulation and dead-space in between would insure soundproofing. Privacy and secrecy were paramount, inherited from mid-Victorian Vienna, and were soon relaxed appropriately as it became clear Americans were not shy about being in psychotherapy and even crowed about it at parties as they compared psychotherapists.

In retrospect, the only time this double-door arrangement proved useful was when I was seeing a patient who was being threatened for wanting to leave the Hell's Angels. During his session, we heard a loud clanking of chains, and my terrified patient declared, "That's Mother coming after me!" The head of the San Francisco chapter was peculiarly called "Mother," a practice that was unfathomable inasmuch as he was a gigantic leathered brute. We heard the outer door open, and as I began to open the inner door, my patient begged me not to do so, fearing for my well-being. Nonetheless, I opened the inner door and stood face-to-face with a baffled hulk that had been thrown completely off balance. Having swung open the outer door and facing yet an inner door, he was too bewildered to argue when I said, "This is a psychotherapy session and you are not allowed to interrupt." He grunted assent, turned around and marched out of the building, chains clanking.

The Yellow Pages of the phonebook promptly and the first time established the designation "psychologists," and with every metropolitan listing there would unfortunately always be a number of quacks. There was no licensure to prevent this and the telephone company refused to screen those seeking listing. This problem was soon addressed by establishing local psychological associations, and the designation (for example) of "Member, San Francisco Bay Area Psychological Association," readily separated the wheat from the chaff in each locale. One established a practice in the usual fashion, speaking to civic and educational institutions, sending out announcements to all physicians, making all the customary rounds, and so forth. There was a shortage of psychotherapists compared to the demand, so practices were soon flourishing, while very prominent psychotherapists maintained months-long waiting lists. I was fortunate at being sought out for spot interviews on the radio in that pre-TV era, and this accorded me unusual exposure to the community. I solved the problem of over-demand by taking on associates to whom I would refer my overflow, thus eliminating any need for a waiting list.

No patient would begin psychotherapy without a battery of interpreted tests, with the "sacred" five being the Wechsler-Bellevue, Rorschach, Thematic Apperception Test, Bender-Gestalt, and Machover Draw-a-Person. Every practicing psychologist had a relationship with a psychiatrist for whom we did psychological testing while they provided services for any of the infrequent medications or hospitalizations that might arise. It must be recalled that in the late 1940s through the 1970s most psychiatrists were still performing mostly psychotherapy. This collaboration was always mutually respectful and totally lacked the professional infighting that is characteristic of today. There was, however, strong resistance by the organization of ApA itself inasmuch as it regarded the rapidly emerging profession of psychology an economic threat.

As part of the therapeutic contract, all patients agreed to pay for any missed sessions that had not been prearranged. There was no third party reimbursement in that early era, so the patient had to cough-up the payment. Also, every patient was required to abide by an agreed upon prearrangement to pay after each session, or monthly. Those of us who sent out monthly statements, this was the task of the therapist's wife as overwhelmingly most of us were male WWII veterans.

Professional liability (malpractice) insurance did not exist until the advent of licensure. All of us practiced with the constant threat that one malpractice judgment would have us paying for life inasmuch as bankruptcy by law excludes malpractice judgments. We assuaged this by meeting regularly as a group that discussed ethics, sound practice, and safeguards. We were so scrupulous, making every disagreement a therapeutic issue for discussion, that lawsuits were rare and even nonexistent. When an occasional malpractice suit occurred we soon learned that it stemmed from patient dissatisfaction with the lack of progress in psychotherapy, expressed in failure to pay the bill. But it was not until the psychologist turned over the account to a collection agency that the patient fought back with a malpractice suit. Consequently we soon learned to never invoke a collection agency, and advised our colleagues to just swallow the unpaid bill.

Play therapy for children was in vogue, pediatricians made frequent referrals, and many psychologists maintained a playroom for that purpose. Psychological testing was a large part of any psychologist's practice, and pediatricians, primary care physicians and psychiatrists all made frequent referrals for testing of their own patients. Our practices were exciting, professionally gratifying, and financially successful. Licensure bureaucracies were nonexistent, there were no knit-picking "guidelines" from the APA, and managed care that was to one day dictate how we practiced was still in the distant future. Psychotherapy was unequivocally the first line intervention in behavioral health. The public adored us as it elevated us to the lofty status of the premier profession. This was truly the Golden Age of Psychotherapy.

# Expanding Psychotherapy to the General Population

Two problems existed and persisted during this era. One was that psychotherapy was sought by the middle and affluent classes, with degree of education highly correlated with the seeking of these services. The working, or so-called blue collar classes, were only slightly represented among those seeking psychotherapy. The second problem was the over-hospitalization of psychotic patients, resulting in the serious over-crowding of our mental state hospitals that provided essentially custodial care.

## The Arrival of Prepaid Mental Health

The first of these problems was addressed by the Kaiser Permanente Health System. In the late 1950s, it began making psychotherapy a covered benefit when referred by a physician. My colleague and I demonstrated (Follette & Cummings, 1967; Cummings & Follette, 1968) through medical cost offset research that psychotherapy was not only economically feasible, but its introduction saved medical/surgical dollars far beyond the cost of providing the behavioral care services. On the basis of this research, I wrote the nation's first comprehensive prepaid psychotherapy insurance benefit in 1959 that became the basis for the healthcare industry to regard psychotherapy as not only feasible, but economically desirable (Cummings & VandenBos, 1981). NIMH was so impressed that it sponsored a number of replications of the Cummings and Follette research that captured the positive attention of third-party payers (Jones & Vischi, 1979).

Following my tenure at Kaiser Permanente, its retrospective findings were spectacularly replicated in the randomized, controlled Hawaii Project that involved the entire Medicaid and federal employee populations (N=130,000) in Hawaii (Cummings, Dorken, Pallak and Henke, 1991; 1993). These two delivery systems (Kaiser Permanente and the Hawaii Project) became the basis for the rapid, widespread extension of health insurance benefits to include mental health, with psychotherapy as the undisputed first line intervention.

## Meeting the Challenge of the Over-Hospitalization of Psychotic Patients

The problem of the over-hospitalization of psychotic patients, along with the serious over-crowding of our state hospitals, was not so deftly resolved. Eventually, it led to deinstitutionalization, and by the 1980s, rendered the street as the de facto mental health hospital, with the prison system not far behind.

In the 1960s and 1970s, NIMH was funding a bold research program known as the Soteria Project in California. Headed and designed by forward thinking NIMH psychiatrist Loren Mosher, the two Soteria Houses, named after the Greek word for "deliverance," were behaviorally-oriented alternatives to hospitalization. In its randomized, controlled research design, every third patient presenting for mental hospitalization in Santa Clara County (California) was remanded instead to one of the Soteria Houses. The program was behaviorally based, using milieu therapy, community self-governance, individual and group psychotherapy, family therapy and other appropriate behavioral techniques, with less than 10% receiving psychotropic medication, and then only for short periods. Additionally, the two-thirds of patients who were committed to the state hospital were transported wearing shackles, while the Soteria patients were transported with no physical restraints by a small, young social worker using her little Volkswagen "beetle."

During three of the dozen years of the Soteria Project, I was privileged to be the director of Palo Alto's prestigious Mental

Research Institute whose staff were the principle investigators and thus administered the Soteria Houses. I was a frequent visitor at the two houses, and although they were both known as Soteria, the second that was opened internally was called Emanon House to differentiate it from its predecessor. On one occasion, I was invited by the patient residents to dinner, but when I arrived at 6:00 p.m. the community was in session deciding what to do with one of the young men who had struck a fellow female patient. As I was not a member of the community, I was excluded; and I cooled my heels until after 11:00 p.m. when the final vote was taken. The decision was made not to expel the perpetrator, who, in exchange, agreed to certain sanctions. This was not an uncommon event, but in all similar such cases the community not only came together, but its decisions were effective.

Most impressive was the ongoing research that revealed the remarkable success of the Soteria program over that of hospitalization for young adult schizophrenics, all without resorting to medications as the treatment. There were impressively fewer relapses, inpatient stay was significantly shorter, and the gainful employment rate after discharge was more than twice that of the state hospitalization experience (Mosher & Hendrix, 2004). In spite of all this, NIMH fired Dr. Mosher and withdrew the project finds, literally in the middle of the night, because as a successful solution to the overcrowding of our state hospitals it was a threat to the fledgling medicalization of mental health that was already underway, and will be discussed later in this chapter.

## Reducing Hospitalization in Mental Health Crises in General

When a patient suffering emotional distress is brought to the emergency room in the middle of the night, the usual procedure is to phone the psychiatrist on call. After a brief discussion with the E.R. physician, the psychiatrist recommends keeping the patient overnight in a holding situation, followed by "I'll be there in the morning." By that time, the patient who has spent the night in a "crazy place" concludes, "I must be crazier than I thought" and projects this self-image. Thus, hospitalization in a psychiatric facility is inevitable.

However, there is another way. The Biodyne Model was founded by me in 1980 as the Biodyne Institute and became a for profit company in 1985. In a simple, but unique procedure that my staff and I developed, a specially trained psychologist, social worker or nurse practitioner will go immediately when called to the E.R. and begins *outpatient* psychotherapy then and there. If the patient responds to outpatient behavioral interventions, he/she obviously does not need to be kept overnight and is sent home with a responsible family member. The patient is seen in the outpatient setting the very next day, with timing that allows the patient to get some sleep, and every successive day until the patient is stabilized. All of this costs but a fraction of what one day of psychiatric hospitalization would cost, and American Biodyne, using this method, was successful in reducing such inpatient care by 90% (Cummings, Cummings & Johnson, 1997). That this simple, effective procedure was never adopted reflects (a) that "medicalized" psychiatrists no longer are trained to do psychotherapy, and (b) the use of non-psychiatric personnel in E.R. coverage is an economic and political threat to the establishment.

## The Medicalization of Mental Health

When psychiatry began in the late 1970s and into the early 1980s to seriously transition from a psychotherapy profession to a medication dispensing practice, the process was formally named "remedicalization" to emphasize the notion that psychiatry was always medical. By the late 1980s, however, the transition was accomplished and the "re" prefix was dropped and is now only a memory to those of us who lived through the process. The term will be recalled when describing the initial formal transition. Of greater importance, however, are the precursors to the process that led up to the formal transition. As used historically in the industry and in this chapter, the term "medicalization" is defined as the process in which psychiatry, and mental health in general, abandoned the concept that emotional and mental conditions are the result of developmental and other untoward experiences for which psychotherapy is the appropriate treatment. Instead, these conditions are attributed to changes in brain chemistry for which psychotropic medications for depression and anxiety (antidepressants and anxiolytic drugs) are the appropriate treatment.

## Deinstitutionalization

In the 1950s, psychiatry discovered Thorazine that it heralded as the "magic bullet" in the treatment of schizophrenia, and would make possible the emptying of our over-crowded mental hospitals. After all, the drug could be prescribed on an outpatient basis, and the movement called deinstitutionalization began in earnest. I was on the staff of Mendocino (California) State Hospital where one of the pivotal researches on Thorazine was conducted by its clinical director, Robert Noce, M.D. In an institution of several thousand court-committed psychotics plus several hundred health staff, it was not possible to hide the shenanigans that went on in this landmark research. The staff was abuzz with the frequent shifting of patients in the experimental (Thorazine) group who were doing poorly to the control group, while patients who were doing well on placebo were reassigned to the experimental group. The staff, who was quite upset over this violation of scientific procedure, took advantage of the fact that "noce" means nut in Italian, and began calling the principle investigator "Doctor

Nut." A group wrote a letter to the funder of the project, but it was ignored, and Robert Noce was given the prestigious Lasker Award for his ostensible landmark research.

Everyone now knows Thorazine was not a magic bullet; deinstitutionalization has been a failure, while the street has become the de facto mental hospital, along with its close cousin, the prison system. For this author, this early experience has inured him to the alarming numbers of bad and even unethical research projects currently being disclosed in psychotropic medicine (Carlat, 2010; Kirsch, 2010).

## The Evolution of the DSM

The American Psychiatric Association's first Diagnostic and Statistical Manual of Mental Health Disorders, or DSM-I, came into being in 1952 and is known colloquially as the "psychiatric bible." Its impetus was the growing number of health insurers and government agencies that were beginning to reimburse for psychotherapy, and they were having difficulty identifying reimbursable conditions inasmuch as every "school" of psychotherapy was using its own esoteric language and diagnostic terminology. Little used at first, over the years it has become not only mandatory for reimbursement, but it is the nomenclature by which government and other agencies collect statistical data on aspects of mental and emotional illness. However, through the years to the present DSM-IV, controversy regarding its efficacy has increased steadily.

## DSM-I: The Age of Anxiety

DSM-I was a relatively succinct and simple document compared to its most recent successors. In the 1950s and 1960s, when psychiatry was still under the influence of European scientific tradition, there was a striving for reasonably accurate diagnoses, as reflected in the DSM-I (Shorter, 2010). Furthermore, it must be remembered, although it has become more difficult to believe in the last two decades, that psychiatry was still psychotherapeutically oriented. "Psychoneurosis" was the principle diagnosis of the day, which simply put, if a patient complained of being "blue. uneasy or generally jumpy, 'nerves' was the common diagnosis. To the psychotherapeutically oriented psychiatrists of the day, 'psychoneurosis' was the equivalent of nerves" (Shorter, 2010, p. 1). There was no reason to delineate this further as both doctor and patient understood "a case of nerves."

In contrast to today's Age of Depression, this was the Age of Anxiety. Two highly regarded and generally read books were Rollo May's *The Meaning of Anxiety* (1950, 1977) and Hans Selye's *Stress* (1956). In coining the term "stressor," Selye added a word universally invoked by psychiatrists and psychologists of the era (Menand, 2010). But then the universal nature of anxiety fostered the fiasco of the earliest psychotropic medications. In 1955, meprobamate with the brand name Milltown was introduced as an anxiolytic, and soon it became the largest selling drug in American history up to that time (Tone, 2009). In fact, it accounted for one third of *all* prescriptions written by American physicians. It is startling to recall that Milltown was soon eclipsed by two other anxiolytics, Librium and Valium, introduced in 1960 and 1963. By 1968, Valium became the most prescribed drug in the Western World, and the stock of its manufacturer, Hoffman-La Roche, increased in 1972 to a whopping $73,000 a share (Tone, 2009).

Marketed with FDA approval as non-addictive, I became alarmed as a legion of patients heavily addicted to these anxiolytics filled my practice. My early attempts to sound an alarm were dismissed by both the manufacturer and the FDA, but by 1980 the research was incontrovertible and the FDA issued a warning label, only the second in history after the fetus crippling drug Thalidomide. The warning stated the stressors of everyday life did not warrant the use of such addictive drugs (Tone, 2009). This example is only the first episode of a continued pattern shown by Big Pharma to underplay research revealing negative side-effects of psychotropic drugs. The crash of Librium and Valium sales marked the end of the Age of Anxiety, but there was an overlap with the introduction of DSM-II.

## DSM-II: A Freudian Document Transforming Personality Disorders into Mental Illnesses

The second DSM was more complicated and it was still based on the concepts put forth by Sigmund Freud and secondly by Adolph Meyer. It was the influence of the latter that along with its psychoanalytic foundation, suddenly Character Disorders were renamed Personality Disorders and made the province of psychiatric treatment. By this arbitrary change in designation a vast population was suddenly catapulted into "treatable" status, a questionable move to this day as the Axis II patients, as they were called, are cluttering our mental health system and edging out treatable Axis I patients. This has been of little concern inasmuch as in the soon-to-be-medicalized system all patients are merely treated with psychotropics.

## DSM-III: The End of Psychopathology

The publication of the third iteration in 1980 brought about a sea change and destined mental health to the eventual crisis in which it now finds itself. With energetic Rene Spitzer at the helm, it sought to solve the problem of reliability so that every practitioner given a set of symptoms would come out with the same diagnosis. In so doing, however, the manual did not address an even greater problem, namely validity, defined as the correspondence of symptoms to organic conditions (Greenberg, 2010; Menand, 2010). In other words, other than diseases the end result was a set of "conditions" or "syndromes" characterized by common signs and symptoms, often loosely woven, whose existence as disease and validity could not be proven.

Spitzer did accomplish one positive reform: he purged the DSM of the Freudian jargon that had plagued the previous editions. In so doing, however, he threw out the baby with the bathwater. Psychoanalysis at least struggled to base itself on psychopathology (i.e., cause and effect), but Spitzer inadvertently omitted psychopathology altogether. Consider where medicine would be without pathophysiology, for it would be exactly where it was a century ago, dealing with conditions and syndromes instead of diseases. Armed with this fallacy, the medicalization of psychiatry leaped forward into the current practice of, for every arbitrary syndrome there is a medication (Kirsch, 2010).

To illustrate further the arbitrary nature of the diagnostic system, DSM-III began the process of "diagnoses by ballot," perfected in the next iteration. Just imagine for one minute if the diagnosis of pancreatic cancer or ovarian cancer was rendered by vote rather than blood tests, imaging or biopsy.

# DSM-IV and IV-T.R.: Our Beleaguered Present

This iteration is comprised of a series of controversial and arbitrary positions that have amplified diagnosis by ballot into a process of DSM committees, often deliberating in secret, voting on adding, subtracting or expanding diagnoses, all in the absence of validity. This DSM has promulgated the Age of Depression similar to the Age of Anxiety, but now with the over-diagnosing of depression for which an ever increasing plethora of antidepressants are being prescribed. With severe side-effects looming, we may be heading for the same train wreck with antidepressants that occurred previously with anxiolytics (Greenberg, 2010; Herzberg, 2008; Kirsch, 2010). In addressing the propensity to prescribe antidepressants for the problems of daily living, Wakefield and Horwitz (2007) deplore the elimination of sadness as a normal and informative emotion in daily living. These same authors have summarized the growing body of literature that reveals the relative ineffectiveness of antidepressants, especially in milder cases, along with the startling array of harmful side-effects, many of them quite serious. Psychiatrist Carlat (2010) concludes flatly that psychotherapy might be more effective and less physically destructive than antidepressants, a position espoused by an ever-increasing number of critics inside and outside the profession (Whitaker, 2010).

## Remedicalization and Medicalization

In the late 1970s the "remedicalization" of psychiatry, a word coined to ostensibly underscore the concept that psychiatry was always part of medicine, but had lost its way into psychotherapy, began in earnest. It vowed to make psychiatry a medication and hospitalization discipline, and psychotherapy ceased to be a part of its residency training. By 1985, American Biodyne was flourishing and was hiring many young psychiatrists to manage medication. Not only had they not received training in psychotherapy, but they also openly disdained it when they referred to it as outmoded "talk therapy." Far too many times, I had to intercede when it was reported psychiatrists were saying to patients, "We used to think that talk therapy was effective, but now we know that these problems result from changes in the chemistry of the brain." When two refused to refrain, they were fired over loud protests that they knew best. Biodyne psychiatrists were forbidden in writing from performing psychotherapy, and one had to be fired because he refused to refrain, stating, "I am a psychiatrist and I can do anything."

This was a transitional time that was often turbulent, but psychologists were oblivious to the implications of what was happening, and instead seemed joyful. They reasoned that with psychiatry abandoning psychotherapy, and with social workers not yet entering private practice in appreciable numbers, psychology had become the premier psychotherapy profession. They scoffed at the possibility that referrals would diminish in favor of medication as they figuratively buried their heads in the sand. They were, in effect, inadvertent participants in the economic disruption that was rapidly overtaking mental health services through five distinct thrusts.

## The Thrust from Organized Psychiatry

The profession of psychiatry has always chafed at the idea it was not really a part of medicine. Originally a neurologist, Freud was chased out of Paris by his colleagues, driving him to Vienna where he established his spectacularly successful psychoanalytic practice. But even at the height of his success, he never forgot what happened; and he was openly oppositional when some of his disciples attempted to make psychoanalysis a part of medicine. As history reveals, this they did with lightening rapidity as soon as the "master" died. Non-physicians were excluded from the institutes of psychoanalysis, and non-physicians holding important posts were rapidly deposed. This is how Siegfried Bernfeld, the psychologist founder of the San Francisco Institute of Psychoanalysis, was summarily stripped of his office, a blow from which he never fully recovered.

Medicine had seemingly discovered a magic bullet in penicillin and subsequent antibiotics, and psychiatry longed to emulate this, setting the stage for the leap into the belief that Thorazine and subsequent medications comprised psychiatry's own magic bullet. Brain chemistry theories involving serotonin and dopamine became pro forma, and psychotherapy, increasingly the province of psychology, was abandoned. The seemingly overnight thrust by which this was accomplished is illustrated by the following. In the late 1970s, the American Psychiatric Association president established a blue-ribbon panel of experts to produce a compendium or manual of accepted, evidence-based psychotherapies. I was the only non-psychiatrist on that panel, and I attended every one of its productive meetings. As it neared the conclusion of its assignment, it was summarily disbanded and its compendium was never published. The era of psychotropic medicine had taken over.

## The Changing of the Guard at NIMH

The National Institute of Mental Health, since its establishment post WWII, had always been congenial to psychosocial research such as the previously discussed Soteria Project. The plunge into medicalization was rapidly occurring in 1979 when as president of the APA, I was desperately trying to warn my unconcerned colleagues of the impending danger. At the same time, I was also director of the Mental Research Institute in Palo Alto, the principle investigator for the Soteria Project. Still called "remedicalization," the process was aggressive and often contentious, and my opposition to it was well-known. Seemingly overnight, the direction of NIMH changed, along with the new appointees heading it as well as ADAMHA (Alcohol, Drug Abuse, and Mental Health Administration, the precursor to the current Substance Abuse and Mental Health Services Administration, or SAMHSA). The latter's new director, Gerald Klerman, was aggressively pushing remedicalization and when he heard that I was in the Rockville Center, a sprawling, ugly series of seemingly endless NIMH buildings. I was there on behalf of Soteria, but I was quickly escorted to Gerry's spacious office on the top floor. He served me afternoon coffee and assorted pastries as we sat on a comfortable sofa and chatted in polite disagreement. At my host's behest, a photographer came in and snapped pictures. The next day a picture appeared in the *Washington Post* with the caption "ADAMHA Chief and APA President Agree on the Future of Mental Health." I was outraged, and repeatedly called Klerman who never returned my calls. This incident is only one illustration of the plethora of unprofessional instances occurring as medicalization was aggressively promoted.

## The Role of the Media

The DSM-III firmly established the concept of medicalization, and no sooner was it published when the ApA's medical director, Melvin Sabshin established a media blitz (Whitaker, 2010). He set out to mobilize the 32,000 psychiatrists and by 1983 as many as thirty books a year were being published heralding the medicalized model. It was about that time that I fortuitously flew across country with Mel and the ApA's chief counsel, Jay Cutler. My company, American Biodyne, was being challenged by the ApA in a number of ways, and this accorded an opportunity for them to state that I was fighting a losing battle as the era of psychotherapy was not only waning, but it would soon be over. The ApA actively courted the press while it trained teams of psychiatrists in such workshops as "How to Survive a Television Interview," and even handed out awards to journalists who wrote stories it liked (Whitaker, 2010, p. 273). All of this was so successful that regularly and with increasing rapidity the media spoke of the "revolution" that was occurring in mental health, all to the benefit of patients and society in general, for the "magic bullet" had been found.

# Big Pharma Cinches the Deal

By the 1980s, the manufacturers of psychotropic medications had fully aligned themselves with the psychiatrists' thrust toward remedicalization. Big Pharma, of course, had the money and the incentive to promote its products, so it is no surprise that it began openly to provide all kinds of stipends to cooperative psychiatrists, as well as to the ApA whose revenues jumped from $10.5 million in 1980 to $21.4 million in 1987. The pharmaceutical companies quickly learned how to effectively turn medical centers into front line publicity churners who were viewed by the public as the "men of science" who were bringing about the revolution that would soon end mental illness (Whitaker, 2010, p. 276).

The extent of the ApA-pharmaceutical partnership was no more demonstrated than in the crass development of teams of "experts" who were not only well-rehearsed, but appeared regularly in media interviews. Any departure from the script resulted not only in being dropped from the team, but all "goodies" promptly stopped coming the offender's way. Add this media blitz to the billions of dollars the pharmaceutical companies spend annually on promoting their products while deemphasizing their side-effects, it is no wonder the American public is only now beginning to become aware of the limitations of the era of medicalization.

The public's propensity for a quick fix certainly increased its susceptibility to the blitz. However, this media campaign would not have been possible were it not for a previous fortuitous event. In a well-meaning change intended to give the public more discretion, the FDA in the 1970s eliminated the distinction between what was termed ethical, or prescription drugs, and over-the-counter, or OTC drugs. Up until that time, only OTC drugs could be advertised to the general public, while ethical drugs could only be marketed to licensed physicians. This distinction led to a plethora of pharmaceutical representatives, commonly known as "detail" men or women, regularly descending on physicians with promotional materials, samples, and gifts for both the doctors and their families. But the kind of constant television, radio and print media advertising that now bombards all of us was not possible. Certainly the ostensibly well-meaning FDA did not anticipate what would occur as the ApA and Big Pharma took advantage of the elimination of this important prohibition.

In its response to Freudian psychoanalysis that put the blame for mental illness on the parents, the National Alliance for the Mentally Ill (NAMI) rejected the psychological origin of schizophrenia and espoused the concept of "brain disease." It eagerly joined the ApA not only in its media blitz, but in lobbying Congress in a concerted effort to promote the brain disease concept. Composed largely of families of schizophrenics, their appeal was regarded as unbiased and salutary by both the Congress and the public.

## Medicalization Completed

Currently 80 to 85% of all psychiatric medications are prescribed by non-psychiatric physicians. This includes antidepressives, anxiolytics and pain killers, and is an outcome predicted three decades ago by psychiatrist Stanley Lesse, long time editor of the *American Journal of Psychotherapy* (Lesse, 1982). The medicalization of psychiatry, Lesse reasoned, would reduce that profession to dull every-fifteen-minute medicine evaluations, rendering it an uninteresting residency and a dull future endeavor for the overwhelming majority of medical school graduates. Additionally, the intuitive (i.e., non-validity) nature of psychiatric diagnoses has suppressed even further the probability that medical school graduates would enter into such a profession in the era of remarkable scientific advances in mainstream medicine. He predicted the current shortage of psychiatrists, along with his stating that primary care physicians would soon become the main pre-scribers of so-called psychiatric medications.

Since patients suffering from anxiety, depression and other forms of emotional distress almost invariably first present themselves to their family physicians and primary care doctors, the fact that these care givers have made psychiatric medication the first line intervention in such cases completes the medical-ization of mental health. Referral for psychotherapy has become a distant second choice. Additionally, family physicians are pre-scribing "off label," defined as prescribing a drug for medical or psychiatric conditions other than the condition approved by the FDA for that particular drug. The majority of such off label pre-scribing is for antidepressants targeting such diverse conditions as obesity, premature ejaculation, shyness, job or marital dissatisfac-tion, teenage rebelliousness, mild compulsive behavior, and poor school grades, all behaviors for which psychotherapy is best suit-ed. Now that family physicians are doing the bulk of psychotropic prescribing, the medicalization of mental health is complete.

Although it is not necessarily so, managed care has con-cluded that medications are cheaper and are also less complicated to administer than psychotherapy. Consequently, the third-party payers have essentially aligned themselves with the medicaliza-tion of psychiatry, and conduct their health plans accordingly.

## Wither and Whither Psychology?

The economics of disruption are a two-way street. As the new replaces the old, there is always a substantial degree of head-in-the-sand behavior by the disrupted. Just as the telegraph indus-try scoffed that the telephone was simply an interesting toy with no future, psychology and the other psychotherapy professions remained in denial over the three decades in which the medical-ization of psychiatry took place. To be sure, a number of positive developments and advances in psychotherapy mark this era. For example: (a) In spite of much initial resistance, evidence-based treatment has finally dominated psychology. (b) Cognitive behavior therapy has developed into the dominant modality, but not without some disadvantages. (c) Psychotherapy has been purged of blaming parents, and especially mothers, for causing schizophrenia and other forms of mental illness.

But these were not sufficient to compensate for the denial of what was forthcoming, and now psychology and other the psychotherapy professions must face the following mistaken notions and behaviors:

- Throughout the medicalization of mental health, organized psychology dodged the issue by insisting psychotherapy is indispensable and will always be the first-line intervention in mental health. Medication is a secondary treatment in severe or infrequent cases. (Note that psychotherapy referrals have declined by 40% and continue to decline.)

- In another head in the sand attitude, it was believed that since psychiatry has abandoned psychotherapy, psychology has become and will remain the premier psychotherapy profession. Social work and counseling will never replace psychology in this role. (Note that master's level practitioners now far out-number psychologists on referral panels, and as much as 80% of psychotherapy is conducted by non-doctoral psychotherapists.)

- Perhaps the most nonsensical position was the following: Healthcare, and especially mental healthcare, are based on the doctor-patient relationship and therefore can never industrialize. This was repeated over two decades by the American Psychological Association in spite of my consistent attempts to warn that soon Wall Street would be dictating our practices if we did not form our own mental health delivery systems (see, for example, Cummings, 1986). After it became a fait accompli, the leadership of the APA spent a decade "exonerating" itself by actively blaming the messenger, and to a lesser extent continues to do so.

- In DSM's purging psychotherapy of psychoanalytic jargon and arrogance, it also discarded all the useful aspects of psychodynamics, thus throwing out the baby with the bathwater. Little by little psychodynamics are creeping back into cognitive therapy by the subterfuge of renaming the techniques, or directly through the work of such bold, articulate psychologists as Shedler (2010).

- From its infancy, clinical psychology distanced itself from mainstream healthcare, and the psychotherapists who followed (counseling, social work practice, MFTs) did the same. Participating as an equal partner in healthcare was disdained as the "medical model," even though today, the rise of nurse practitioners, podiatrists, and other treatment disciplines has long ago changed this to the "healthcare model." To this day, our creation of two separate silos, health and mental health, plagues us as we are often overlooked by policy makers, healthcare companies and the general public, resulting in our getting the crumbs when budgets are constructed.

- The first behavior/primary care project in which behavioral care providers (BCPs) worked side by side with primary care providers (PCPs) I was privileged to establish in 1963, and its success was immediate in terms of both medical and psychotherapeutic results. Nonetheless, the APA rejected the model for 46 years, finally adopting it as policy in 2009 after it had been adopted by the U.S. Air Force, several V.A. hospitals, and parts of TriCare. So far, only a few such integrated projects exist in non-government centers, mostly because psychologists have not been trained to create such delivery systems. Most of the efforts that pass for integrated behavioral/primary care are simply singular interventions such as obesity or depression programs that have been parachuted into a traditional health setting and are pawned off as full integration.

- Psychotherapists have distinguished themselves as economic illiterates, thus they were unable to recognize the egregious economic thrusts that were being promulgated in the medicalization of mental health. There seems to be an antipathy among psychotherapists in regard to economics as if the business of succeeding financially and that of "doing good" are somehow incompatible. Perhaps our colleagues can begin by monthly balancing their personal checkbooks. In a recent anecdotal survey, I was startled at the number of psychotherapists who seldom if ever reconcile their own personal bank accounts, while blindly accepting their bank's balance sheet at the end of every month.

- Well over a decade ago, practitioners within the APA began to actively work toward prescription authority for psychologists specially trained in psychopharmacology. This set off a firestorm, splitting the organization into two militant camps. Those favoring what came to be known as RxP were mostly fulltime practitioners, while those vehemently opposing essentially had full or part-time academic appointments. Only two states, Louisiana and New Mexico, have enacted such legislation, while psychologists in the military have been prescribing successfully for a number of years. The controversy has somewhat subsided, but largely because RxP has stalled. There have been unfortunate incidents in which psychologists have last-minute openly lobbied against RxP bills that were within the reach of passage, only widening the rift.

- Now that psychiatry has become solely a medication profession, there is a need for a mental health profession that has prescription authority while mostly performing psychotherapy. The advantage is that prescription authority enables the practitioner to take patients off of medication as well. It is understandable why psychiatry would oppose such competition, but why academic psychologists oppose RxP is an enigma that must be left to another discussion.

Our national organizations (American Psychological Association, National Association of Social Work, American Counseling Association, and American Marriage and Family Therapy Association) are now aware there are problems as they have literally been thrown in their faces, but they remain bereft of much needed innovative solutions. Splinter organizations such as the aggressive, vocal, five-year-old National Association of Professional Psychology Providers (www.NAPPP.org) is spearheading change largely because it is first and solely a practitioner organization, while our main-line associations are largely controlled by academics prone to cogitate, but not innovate.

## Is Another Disruption on the Way?

There is a mounting array of research demonstrating the ineffectiveness of psychiatric medications along with their serious side-effects, accompanied by a plethora of class action lawsuits brought against the manufacturers. The exposing of the unethical closeness of psychiatrists with Big Pharma, indications of highly questionable research, revelations of scientific publications ghost-written by the industry rather than by the alleged author, along with a host of other troublesome disclosures are coming to the attention of the general public. Furthermore, that non-psychiatric physicians are prescribing as much as 80% of the psychiatric medication is a problem of significant proportion. Are these indicating the emergence of another disruption, perhaps returning psychotherapy to its place as the first line intervention in behavioral care? This and related issues are the subject of the succeeding chapters.

# References

Carlat, D.J. (2010). *Unhinged: The trouble with psychiatry – A doctor's revelations about a Profession in crisis.* New York: Free Press.

Christensen, C.M., with Grossman, J.H. & Hwang, J. (2009). *The innovator's prescription: A disruptive solution for healthcare.* New York: McGraw Hill.

Cummings, N.A. (1986). The dismantling of our health system: Strategies for survival of psychological practice. *American Psychologist, 41,* 426-431.

Cummings, N.A. & Follette, W.T. (1968). Psychiatric services and medical utilization in a prepaid health plan setting: Part 2. *Medical Care, 6,* 31-41.

Cummings, N.A., Cummings, J.L., & Johnson, J.N. (1997) (Eds.).*Behavioral health in primary care: A guide for clinical integration.* Madison, CT: Psychosocial Press.

Cummings, N.A., Dorken, H., Pallak, M.S., & Henke, C.J. (1991). The impact of psychological intervention on healthcare costs and utilization. The Hawaii Medicaid Project. *HCFA Contract Report #11-C-983344/9.*

Cummings, N.A., Dorken, H., Pallak, M.S., & Henke, C.J. (1993). The impact of psychological intervention on healthcare costs and utilization: The Hawaii Medicaid Project. In N.A. Cummings & M.S. Pallak (Eds.), *Medicaid, managed behavioral health and implications for public policy.* (pp. 3-23), Vol. 2: Healthcare and utilization cost series. South San Francisco, CA: Foundation for Behavioral Health.

Follette, W.T. & Cummings, N.A. (1967). Psychiatric services and medical utilization in a prepaid health plan setting. *Medical Care, 5,* 25-35.

Greenberg, G. (2010). *Manufacturing depression.* New York: Simon and Schuster.

Herzberg, D. (2008). *Happy pills in America.* Baltimore: Johns Hopkins University Press.

Jones, K.R. & Vischi, T.R. (1979). The impact of alcohol, drug abuse, and mental health treatment on medical care utilization: A review of the research literature. *Medical Care, 17,* (suppl.), 43-131.

Kirsch, I. (2010).*The emperor's new drugs.* New York: Basic Books.

Lesse, S. (1982).The uncertain future of clinical psychiatry. *American Journal of Psychotherapy,* 37(2), 306-312.

May, R. (1950).*The meaning of anxiety.* New York: Norton (Rev. Ed. 1977).

Menand, L. (2010). Can psychiatry be a science? *New Yorker,* March 10: http://www.newyorker.com/arts/critics/2010/03/01/100301crat_ atlargw.menand?curr

Mosher, L.R. & Hendrix, V., with Fort, D.C. (2004). *Soteria: Through madness to deliverance.* Bloomington, IN: Xlibris.

Selye, H. (1956). *Stress.* New York: McGraw-Hill.

Shedler, J. (2010). The efficacy of psychodynamic psychotherapy. *American Psychologist,* 65(2), 98-109.

Shorter, E. (2010). Why psychiatry needs therapy. *Wall Street Journal (WSJ.com):* http://online.Wsj.com/article_email?S BG10001424052748704570081370022760116

Tone, A. (2009). *The age of anxiety: A history of America's turbulent affair with tranquilizers.* New York: Basic Books.

Wakefield, J. & Horowitz, A. (2007).*The loss of sadness.* Piscataway, NJ: Rutgers University Press.

Whitaker, R. (2010). *Anatomy of an Epidemic.* New York: Crown.

Wright, R.H. & Cummings, N.A. (Eds.) (2001).The practice of psychology: The battle for Professionalism. Phoenix, AZ: Zeig, Tucker and Theisen.

Chapter 2
# Renewing the Clinical Relationship
*(Transcribed by permission from the video recording of the presentation)*

*David Healy, M.D.*

Nick outlined a problem that we all have, and it's a problem where, as he put it out to you, it is clear that almost whatever we do we seem to make the problem worse. Why do the forms of treatment that seem to work and the ones that seem to be the right kind of treatments to offer, get closed down even when they have got data in their favor? So I'm hoping to try to pick up on that, but hoping also to do a little bit more. For years and years and years, I have been giving talks and writing books and giving lectures on these issues, and it seems to me that almost everything I have done in trying to describe the problem has made things worse, not better. The ultimate sad point of this came home to me a few years ago. After I had written the book, *Let Them Eat Prozac,* I met the person who was responsible for the marketing of Prozac in the United Kingdom. She came up to me and said, "Oh, you're David Healy. I'm so pleased to meet you. You're doing more for the sales of Prozac in the U.K. than anyone else."

So we have a real problem here, as the system we seem to be up against is some kind of strong system that needs all of us to protest. I shall try to outline the nature of the system, but the system needs people to protest. It needs Nick to protest and David to protest and Bob to protest and me to protest and all of you, for actually you are helping the system when you just say, "Aren't things awful?" We need to do more than say, "Aren't things awful?" We need to find a way out of the system.

So ultimately I'm going to pose a big question, and I am here looking for answers, and I am hoping that you are all going to be able to help me find the answer. I don't have the answer. At least, I have what I think may be a hint of an answer, but I am hoping all of you will be able to come onboard and help me sort out and work out how we go forward from here.

As I lay out this problem, I am hoping you will not just have questions, but that you will be offering answers. There is one more reason why you need to engage with this. As Nick said, this is not about mental healthcare; this is about all of healthcare. The problems you are looking at now at this meeting are ones you have possibly approached in terms of your job as a therapist. What are the problems for a therapist? What are the opportunities for being able to get work? What are the issues about getting reimbursed? What's happening to the market?

What I want you to realize, however, is that you are two people. Yes, each of you are two people. You have a job: You do therapy. But you are also at some point going to be a patient. For some the healthcare problem is there, but not personal. As a patient, however, you are trapped in the system and you are going to have problems of just the kind that I am going to outline here. So as therapists, you need to find an answer to the problems, but also as potential patients, you need to find an answer, too.

Now part of the problem is this: Nick ended by saying that there has recently been a law case. There are things that are happening that are good. There are legal cases that bring a whole range of things to light. They bring to light the fact that there are an awful lot of articles being ghostwritten. They bring to light other facts, such as the ways that the pharmaceutical companies market drugs to us. And there is a group of people, again like Nick and David and me and Bob and others whom I meet in meetings like this in which all of us get the feeling at times that things are moving in the right direction. We get a buzz from the gathering like this as we think; here we are, all on the same page. And we think if all of us are on the same page, we can make a difference. But are things getting better?

Nick has referred in our talks to the law suit following the birth defects resulting from the prescribing of Paxil, an antidepressant, to pregnant woman. I was an expert witness in that trial. It was an extraordinary case that showed just how much the company had gone to deliberately market antidepressants to women of childbearing years, knowing that the drug they were marketing could cause women to become physically hooked to it. And also knowing that it doubles the rate of birth defects, doubles the rate of miscarriages, and it doubles the rate of voluntary terminations when you are on the drug. It causes all sorts of other problems to the child when it is born, and quite possibly causes children to be behaviorally retarded later in life. Knowing all these things, the drug was still aggressively marketed.

The impact of that case, I think, has been nil even though the company lost. The media barely covered it, and even now that all of the information has come out and is in the public domain, what the company did is known by only a few people. It does not get out there to the general public and it does not make a difference in the healthcare you get. And that's the way things have been. From the first S.S.R.I. psoriasis case that hit the media to a degree, to the most recent birth defect case that hardly hit the media at all, we are up against a system that closes down the kinds of information that are inconvenient to the system.

It does more. As Nick outlined very well, a key point is that forty years ago the patients were very visible to the person treating them. Clinical care was all about a patient who had a problem or thought they had a problem who came along to a person like you or Nick or me or whoever, asking for help, and care was all about the help we gave to them. You could see the patient there in front of you. The problem now is most doctors cannot see the patient anymore. It is a bit like this: They see the chair, but they don't see the patient. The data that run the system in which they work, be it the HMO or the healthcare group in which they work, dictates the kind of care they give, almost regardless of the person there in front of them. Your capacity to have any clinical discretion is terribly limited, and if you stray from what the people who employ you say you can do, you run an increasing risk these days of losing your job. You are given clinical trial data, but this is data on hundreds of people that gives you average data about things, not the kind of data often that you need for the person in front of you.

Orthodox medicine is in a crisis rather like the situation the Catholic Church was in 10 years ago because of the sex abuse scandals. There is a profound credibility problem and medicine, in contrast to the Church, who has addressed its credibility gap, is not coming to grips with its own credibility problem. They say they are, but they are not.

Now you may think this is fairly fanciful and does not apply to any of you, for if you had been there when children were being abused by priests in the Church, you would have spoken out. This is the past, the convenient past. But of course children here in the United States in foster care are being abused. Almost all of them are referred to psychiatrists. Almost all of them end up on meds. Almost *all* of them end up two to three hundred pounds in weight. This is as bad as the abuse that was happening in the Catholic Church, and may still be happening in the Catholic Church. Where are you? Have any of you or any of us done anything about this? I am not sure we have. So, while it is not a convenient image from the past it is an image about where we are all now. It is not a problem just for medicine, but for you and me as well.

## The Problem of Conflict of Interest

It is a problem when doctors get paid by the pharmaceutical industry to give lectures, to run clinical trials, to attend professional meetings and to ostensibly write scientific articles that are actually ghostwritten by the industry. They are often paid huge amounts of money, and the argument is that if only they were not paid this money, everything would be okay. Journals, universities and everybody else goes around these days trying to make conflict-of-interest kinds of policies, believing that if they can just get people to adhere to these, everything will be okay. Well, this is not the problem. This is a convenient myth that suits the interests of the pharmaceutical industry. They want you to think that the problem is a few rotten apples in the barrel, whereas the problem is the barrel. And that's what I hope to try to persuade you.

## The Problem of the Patent

Now, there are a few aspects to the problem that we cannot change quickly, but I just need to put them on the map so that you are aware of them. It is only after I get through this part that we will get into things you can change. The first aspect to the problem is that the drugs that you have available here in the U.S.

and worldwide these days are available under product patents. Let me explain what this is to you.

In the case of a drug like Prozac, for example, the way the system works is that the company that makes Prozac gets to hold the patent on it. Back in 1962, this issue was being reviewed in the United States because the different countries around the world had different approaches to the patenting of drugs. The Germans used what were called "process patents"; that is, if one company made Prozac, they could have the patent on it, but if a different company could make the same drug in a different way, they could also hold a patent on it. So you did not have the kind of system where only one company could hold the patent on a drug. So, when this was being reviewed by the U.S. Senate in 1961–62 there were fifty-five countries in the world that have products patent systems and one-hundred twenty-three that have process patents. The average price of drugs in the countries that have products patent systems is fifty-five to two-hundred eighty-seven times higher than in countries that have process patents, and the countries that have product patent systems like the U.S., produce less new drugs than the countries like Germany that operate a process patent system. What are we going to do? What is the obvious logical way forward? And the answer that the committee came up with was, well, we are going to stick to products patents. What they did not say was they were going to persuade the rest of the world to switch from process patents to product patents. They succeeded in doing so in the 1960s and 1970s, for by accomplishing this in the United Kingdom, Germany, and Japan, as the three primary nations needed, and they created a condition where drug companies can make blockbuster drugs.

If you are the only person that can hold a patent on a drug worldwide, you have the conditions that mean you can market the hell out of this drug and really make a fortune from it. If you have a different system, where other companies can make the same drug, you cannot make the same profits out of your drug. You are not going to invest the same amount of money in trying to hype up the benefit of this drug, because you may be just making the market for one of the other companies.

By the early 1980s most of the Western world had changed to a product patent kind of system. In 1961 to 1962, a key drug disaster occurred in the United States and the U.S. Senate was looking for a way to make certain this did not happen again, so they decided to stick with products patents to assure this. The irony of the situation will become clear as I explain, but what they did was to produce a system where it became worthwhile for the pharmaceutical companies to make blockbuster drugs, and the first of these came on stream in the mid '80s. This was a drug, created by GlaxoSmithKline (now GSK) to treat ulcers, that was making an incredible amount of money when a guy in Perth, Australia discovered that antibiotics help and can cure ulcers inasmuch as they are caused by a virus. Because you don't need to give the GSK drug now for life, the company tried to close his research down. So you had a system where the company is making so much money out of the drug, they do not want to hear what the real answer to the problem is.

Prozac came on stream a few years later, and by this time companies are making roughly 10–15% of their profit from blockbuster drugs, which they had not ever done before. The definition of a "blockbuster drug" is one that earns a billion dollars a year or more. Lipitor is the one that earned the most. At its peak, it was earning for Pfizer $13 billion a year for a drug they did not discover and they did not make. They brought it in and just marketed it extraordinarily successfully. As these companies have become better and better at marketing, they have become poorer and poorer at making new drugs of the kinds that we actually need. We are at the point where these drugs are now worth more than their weight in gold to the pharmaceutical industry.

There was a big fuss about a hundred years ago over the patent medicines and the nostrums that were being sold over the counter. In that era, drinks like Coca-Cola actually contained cocaine and 7-Up contained lithium. There was a big concern that these drugs were not only being sold over the counter, but the markup on them was 500%. Can you believe it? The raw ingredient of the drug whatever it might be, cost maybe a cent or two to make and they were charging a dollar. Today the markup for Lipitor and Prozac is 2500%, and there are no complaints. This creates a condition in which fate of the companies hinges on a few drugs that they have rather than a portfolio of drugs. And if the fate of these companies hinges on a few drugs, they cannot let these drugs go down. They are going to hype the benefits of the drugs as much as possible before the patent expires. You are going to hear these drugs are the cure for everything. They are also going to hide the hazards. This is an issue for each of you as patients. Every single drug you are on, whether for asthma or your gut, for hypertension or for diabetes, the hazards are being hidden from you.

## Prescription Authority

There is a further aspect to the problem that cannot be changed in a hurry. Drugs that a woman may be taking by choice such as birth control pills because it is her body and her decision nonetheless require a prescription. The prescription only status of drugs was introduced in 1914 as part of the war on drugs. At that time, this authority was over opiates and cocaine, and although one could certainly buy these drugs without a prescription, many people preferred the physician's judgment as to the safety of a prescription over a non-prescription, believing there is a reasonable chance that this is a useful thing to take.

Prescription-only status was extended to a whole raft of new drugs that came on stream, and these new drugs often worked better in ways older drugs had not. They worked to help cure disease, but because they worked, they also caused harm. Up until then there had been no reason to write a book about the side-effects of drugs, and these books began appearing in 1951. Against such a background came a wave of concern and also skepticism about the pharmaceutical industry, so it was concluded that it would be a good idea to make these new drugs available only by prescription as doctors would know best.

A lot of people here in the U.S. in particular, in a way that might seem inconceivable to you now, protested saying that a system designed for addicts should not be extended to citizens of a free county. You would not get an awful lot of people thinking that was the right way forward now.

## The Stockholm Syndrome

In 1962, because of a drug disaster that you are going to hear more about later in this chapter, the FDA decided to continue with prescription-only status for new drugs because as doctors were skeptical about drugs. Physicians should be the ones who decided how drugs should be administered and to whom and for what conditions. The public agreed that doctors are the people who could get the information out from pharmaceutical industries about what the true risks of these drugs were in a way that you or I could not. And this created a new problem. This created the conditions for the Stockholm syndrome, a clinical condition that you may have heard about, but I will say that it applies in spades to people who are taking drugs on prescription-only and it applies to the prescribers also.

What is the Stockholm syndrome? Well, for those of you that do not know, it is the following. There was a bank in Sweden in which in 1973 a group of armed raiders broke into and held the bank staff hostage for five days. There was a siege. Ultimately, the staff of the bank got out okay, but when interviewed by a stunned media afterwards, there was a universally unexpected outcome to all of this that was: They said, no, the guys that held us hostage with guns and all that were really nice guys. You know, we kind of approve of what they were doing and they were just nice people and they treated us well. And the media and the outside world were intrigued, asking what's going on here? If I were held hostage in a bank, I would be furious with these people who held me hostage. The hostages almost looked as if they were brainwashed. That led to descriptions of this syndrome that seems to come about when you are isolated, when there is a threat to your life and when the captor, or the person who controls the way out, is kind to you.

The implication here is that if you are ill, you are isolated. If you are ill, there is a threat to your life and your doctor is in the business of being kind to you. He or she wants to help you. You have got the perfect conditions for Stockholm syndrome, the kinds of conditions that mean that when you are there being held hostage in the bank, you are not going to be angry with these guys; you are not going to tell them how you really feel. When you are on a drug, you are not going to report the problems you are having on the drug. You do not want your captor to be unhappy. I mean, he is, after all, your way out. Your key job if you are having problems on drugs is not to let him or her know about the problem you are having; your key job is to get out and the doctor is the way out and you want to keep that doctor happy.

There are various ways to frame this, but one is called the "Triangle of Karpman" that operates in all of us. If you take a transactional approach towards these issues, you say that in each of us there is a persecutor and a victim and a savior. Within the health field, anyone who raises hazards about drugs as I do is viewed as the persecutor and the patient is the victim. The people who say, you don't want to believe the black box warnings on drugs that say they are risky and causing more harm than good, are the persecutors. The guys who say that drugs work and have no problems, they view themselves as being the patient's savior. Just what, then, is the right way to describe the dynamics that happen in clinical care? The one key thing you need to know about all this is that your doctor is trained to prescribe, but has never been trained to know that the person receiving the prescription is in a hostage-like situation. And the doctor has no idea how to undo this, as there is no idea about what may be getting in the way of your letting him or her know about the problems that you are having. So how do we undo that?

## Controlled Trials as the Answer?

Now here is the bit of the problem. They are actually two bits that are hard for us to change, but you need to know they are there. Here is the bit of the problem that we can begin to change. There was a drug disaster in 1962, and the drug that caused the problems, was called Thalidomide. It led to children being born without limbs, with heart defects and things like that. In Europe, the drug had been available over-the-counter for treating nausea in pregnancy. Because of the side-effects, one response available to the FDA was to make drugs available on prescription-only. Of course, it was in Europe and not here, where the problems were raised first, and it was in Europe where doctors did not make a living out of this drug so that they were able to recognize the problem. Unlike Paxil, which causes the same problems and is available on prescription-only here in the U.S. and where doctors do not concede that it can cause birth defects. One of the answers to the problem from the FDA's point of view was to introduce control trials, or RCTs. Only if we can show that the treatments that come on the market work, if they go through controlled trials and have been shown to work and if we ensure that only drugs are available that have been shown to work, then everything will be okay, won't it? Well, before 1962, there had been only one drug that had been through a placebo-controlled trial before it was about to come on the market—only one. And the placebo controlled trial for this drug showed that it worked wonderfully effectively as an aid to sleep and was free of side effects. Do you know what that drug was? Can you guess? Or is the answer too shocking? Thalidomide. The system we put in place to ensure that thalidomide does not happen again is a system through which thalidomide sailed beautifully through the system. So if you think we are being protective, think again.

Where are we now that controlled trials have become the answer to the problem? If we believe that if everything is run through controlled trials, there will not be a hazard and we will have drugs that work, let's look at the controlled trial that deserves to be labeled one of the most famous in all of medicine: Cipriani, Furukawa, Salanti, et al (2009). There is a huge authorship of twenty-two odd authors, of which only three are listed here, but this article appears in the journal with the highest impact factor in the field of child psychiatry. These findings are summarized in Figures 1 and 2, and this research is known in the medical literature as Study 329. Figure 1 lists the studies as reported in the journal article, purporting that of the fifty-one trials, all but three were positive. In contrast, Figure 2 gives the breakdown as seen by the FDA, revealing that in actuality thirty-six of seventy-four trials were not positive. It says, as just one example, that "Paxil works wonderfully well for children who are depressed" and it is free of both problems and side effects. Doctors reading an article like this cannot help but be impressed with authors who are huge names in the field publishing in a journal of this stature. They will likely conclude that if this article says that this drug works well, we should be using it. Children who are unhappy, miserable and may be depressed, even if we are not absolutely sure they are depressed. If there is a good chance that they are depressed and we leave it untreated, they are going to go on to suicide, alcoholism , drug abuse, divorce, and even failed careers. After all, this drug is harmless. Giving this antidepressant is just like giving a vitamin, so hey, let's give it.

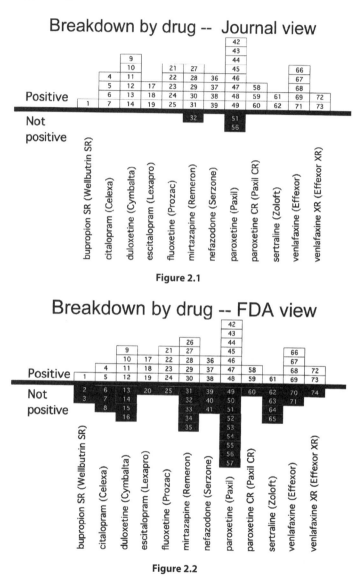

Figure 2.1

Figure 2.2

However, the introduction of Paxil by SmithKlineBeecham in 1998 and released in 2001 (Keller, Ryan and Stobler, et
al., 2001), and which data are included in Study 329, revealed
more non-positive than positive data. So the company concluded it
was risky to show these data to the FDA as it might well conclude
that a drug that did not work for teenagers would likely not work
for adults. So only the positive data were shown to the FDA by the
makers of Paxil as SmithKlineBeecham had concluded it would
be risky for the rest of the world to see all these data. This was the
format subsequently adopted by Study 329. As can be seen in Figure 2, which includes the same data as in the 1998 study, the total,
over-all results show that part of the document pertaining to Paxil
shows the drug does not work. No wonder GlaxoSmithKline, the
successor to SmithKlineBeecham, concluded it was risky for the
company to show the data to the FDA, inasmuch as that agency
might be concerned if it got to see all of this, to say nothing of
the risk if the rest of the world were see the data as well. They
might ask why doctors are giving this drug to adults if the drug
did not work for teenagers. Might it not work for adults either? So
the whole thing was risky all around, and they decided that they
were not going to give the data to the FDA. What they were going to do is to pick the good bits of the data out of Study 329 and
publish those, and that is what you have got in the previous article
shown in Figure 1. You have got the good bits of the data and you
do not have all of the data. No one has access to—or had at that
stage—access to all of the data. You have also seen the authorship line, but what you did not see was the author, Sally Laden.
She is not listed on the authorship line. This is an email from the
point person within SmithKlineBeecham to the author of the article, saying: You know, Sally, you've done awfully well hiding
the serious adverse events in this trial. I mean, I know the serious
adverse events, and the investigators, the people who later end up
as the authors on the authorship line, haven't raised an issue. They

have seen a draft of the article at this point. They have not raised an issue saying, "Hey, look, what about the children who became suicidal? They have just seen a draft of the article. They may or may not have read the draft of the article, but they have not raised any issues. But even I in the company, knowing what I know about this trial, am feeling a little bit uncomfortable here.

Ultimately it becomes clear, because of the document that you have seen there earlier, which wends its way to New York State, and New York State decides to sue GlaxoSmithKline (GSK) based on the fact that what you have got here is fraudulent marketing, that there are an awful lot of children who were given it even though the drug at this stage has not been so approved by FDA."

Later, if New York State does sue the company, it is clear that the drug is not going to be approved by FDA, but hundreds of thousands of kids are already on this drug thanks to an article that appears in the high-impact doctor journal with great authors on it. I mean to say, this is why doctors actually prescribe. They do not prescribe because they are paid money, are brought to the Caribbean, or have pretty women or men come around and leave free kind of samples of the drug. If you asked them why they prescribed it, they say they follow the evidence, and the company is in the business of trying to make sure that the evidence looks just the right way for them. So ultimately what you have got is an awful lot of children put on the drug because of this article, after which New York State decides to sue the company to get the back the money that it paid out for the scripts of this drug. They were being sued for fraud, and not surprisingly the company agreed to settle. As part of the settlement, they handed over a large amount of money and agreed to post the results of the clinical trials they have done on the company website. The world thinks this is great. We have got the pharmaceutical companies now publishing all of the reports from all of the trials that they do on the company website; isn't this great progress?

If you look at the journal itself in which the article came out, the editor of the journal has been approached by a journalist who is asking, "Do you have any regrets about publishing the study?" And the answer is, "I have no regrets at all," and, "Are you aware that this study was ghostwritten? What do you think about this?" And the answer is, "Well, you know, so what? Ghostwriters write awfully well at times and the fact that one person puts the words together one way as opposed to a different way may be a good or bad thing, et cetera, et cetera, et cetera. He conceded this woman is shameless on the issue. Okay? Efforts have been made to get the journal to retract the article, and they point blank refuse. This means that when anybody is drawing up guidelines on the treatment of children who are depressed or anxious, if they do not know the inside story here, they are going to look at the published literature and they are going to download this article and it is going to show Paxil is extremely good for treating children who are depressed and they are going to recommend the use of Paxil for children who are depressed.

## The Published Literature

Nothing seems to be able to change that. But is this is an extraordinary situation? Is it just a strange state of affairs? Is it plain weird or is it the kind of thing that applies to any other drugs that you may end up on, for instance, for your husbands or wives or children or parents? Well, Erick Turner produced an important piece of work three to four years ago while working in the FDA as he was aware of all the trials that had gone to the FDA on the antidepressant drugs that are on the market currently. In regard to all the drugs, he found that the published literature that came out in bringing them to market were positive in beating the placebo.

For example, let's look at Zoloft. There were only two trials, but they were both positive, a 100% positive outcome for this drug. Okay? Now, there are groups of people in place who review the data on the drugs that you or I might take, and this is not just for antidepressants, it is not just mental health, it is for drugs such as statins that are given for diabetes. But it is for any drugs you or your husbands or wives or parents or children could be on. The same applies. There are all sorts of groups who review the published literature and come to views about what is the best drug to use. What are the ones that are reasonably safe and what ones should you maybe steer clear of? And in the case of groups reviewing the antidepressants, there is one group in particular, the Cochran Review Center of which I'm sure you have heard. They painstakingly search for all of the published articles. For instance, they do really good things such as in the case of an antipsychotic like Zyprexa. They are the ones that found there were two-hundred thirty-four publications on this antipsychotic drug four to five years ago, but there were actually only four trials. Two hundred thirty-four publications sounds great, a lot of evidence on this drug, but only four trials, and none of the two-hundred thirty-four publications listed the raised cholesterol levels that the drug causes. It raises them more than any other drug in medicine. None of them give you the data on the raised blood sugars that it causes, and none of them give you the data on the rates at which people go on to commit suicide, yielding perhaps the highest suicide rate in clinical trial history. None of the two-hundred thirty-four publications give you this at all, which is interesting.

Anyway, let's get back to the antidepressants, such as Zoloft. The Cochran reviews of the publication in *Lancet,* an extremely good journal, found the conclusion that if you are going to go on an antidepressant, what you want is Zoloft. Tell your doctor to give you Zoloft. It is the one based on the published literature that is the best. However, Erick Turner went a little bit further, which he could do because he knew where the corpses were. He knew that there had been more trials that went in to FDA than the published literature hinted at, and when you get all of the trials of these drugs, what you get is a picture of all the negative studies on these drugs. You see that over 40% of the studies were negative. And if you look farther for the worst drug, thanks to the Cochran review that gives access to all of these files, you would find that going to pick out the worst drug, the antidepressant you would pick is Zoloft because only one of the five trials that were done was positive. And the Cochrane studies reveal much more. There are an awful lot of trials that are negative that do not get published, but, furthermore, there are trials that are negative that do get published, but have become positive by the time they are published, just like Study 329, which is a negative trial but gets transformed into one that is positive.

So, Erick went a little further and described a group of other trials that had been published as being positive that FDA had actually regarded as being negative. And there is a group of different ways to do it. Let me hop for a second from the antidepressants for a moment. Many of you will have patients who are on a mood stabilizer for bipolar disorder, and one of the ones that is being pushed very heavily at the moment is Abilify. Abilify is an extraordinary drug that I could tell you an awful lot about, but the trial that got FDA approval for it was one where the results from all of the centers, bar one, actually suggested that the drug did not work at all. It was only on the basis that the trial included one center down in Mexico that had totally different results to anywhere else that you could show a marginal difference between the drug and placebo. And based on this, FDA approved it for the maintenance treatment of bipolar disorder. As Erick points out, what you have got the companies doing is things like that, but the other way around: If there is one center that does not produce the right results, somehow that gets dropped out of the frame and they just handle the results of the five centers that have produced the good results, or they change the endpoint.

In the case of Study 329, if you looked closely at it, the primary endpoint was one in which the drug failed. But what gets written up are the data in terms of the other rating scales that were used. This is what is used to bring out the point or to make the case that the drug worked. So there is a range of tricks that the companies can use to portray their drug in a positive light.

What are the consequences of this in terms of hiding the adverse effects of drugs? In the case of the antidepressants, what happens in the clinical trials is, you get people who have been removed from the drug they were on before, and then they begin the clinical trial proper. To repeat, they get removed from the prior drug they were on before they go into the trial proper that begins later. It is now clear that when you remove people from a previous drug they were on, they often go into withdrawal, and an awful lot of people go on actually to a suicidal act. This is almost the riskiest part of treatment. The rates at which people go on actually to a suicidal act in clinical trials are higher during the washout phase. Later on, when they run the trials proper for Prozac, Zoloft, and Paxil, you have suicides and the suicidal acts on the drug down, and then you also have the suicides and the suicidal acts on the placebo. But there are more suicides and suicidal acts happening on the active drug than on the placebo, partly because there were more people put on the active drug than on the placebo, but the data would look awfully bad for the companies. So it had to be handled in any of the publications you see in the literature, almost all of which are ghostwritten these days.

## Ghostwriting

When I talk about articles being ghostwritten, people try to estimate what proportion of the literature is ghostwritten these days for Lipitor, Avandia, and Advert—forget Prozac for the moment—but for all of these drugs, what proportion of the literature on drugs do you think is ghostwritten. Can we take an estimate? How many people think half of the literature on these drugs is ghostwritten? A bit higher, please. Twenty-five percent ghostwritten? 75% ghostwritten? Well, it is awfully hard to work this out. Let me ask the question in a slightly different way and see if we get the same answers. If published trials are the main tools that a pharmaceutical company uses to market the product, then what is in the trial has to be favorable. What proportion of these trials do you think the pharmaceutical industry will let out of their control, will let someone else write up? Ten percent? Twenty percent? Zero percent? Well, there is close to incontrovertible evidence that at least 50-odd percent or more have been ghostwritten.

The problem we have that they write the first draft and it goes out to the authors whose names end up on it. These authors have five days to get back, and the article that ends up in print is unchanged word for word; there is not a single word changed. You still get the authors of these articles saying, "No, the ghostwriters didn't write this; I wrote this article." So you are up against a problem trying to conclude whether an article like that is ghostwritten or not. But the agency that writes the article writes the article, and the finished (published) product is 100% the same, except for ones that added the authors' declaration that they were supported by a grant from the NIH, or some such agency. In such cases your tax dollars pay not only for the work, but also to ghostwrite the article. Nonetheless you will still get the response, "No, I wrote this article." So it can be hard to pin it all down.

So here is what happened to suicidal acts in the published literature, and this is most interesting. The rationale for this is: Well, these people have been removed from the previous drug that is just the same as being on placebo. Isn't it? So we just move all these data, which is what GlaxoSmithKline did. But one guy in the placebo group, for example, who was followed after the clinical trial was over, did not seem quite right. So his doctor put him on Prozac, and a week or two after he is on Prozac, he committed suicide. He becomes a placebo suicide! So it is things like this that are being written up by the ghostwriters who actually write the material.

## Posting of Clinical Trials on the Web

So let's move on. But of course, as you know, that is all in the past tense, for ostensibly everything has been put right because the companies now post all the clinical trials up on the web. Well, not so. When the data from all the trials are systematically posted on the web as evidence there is no longer a problem anymore, but there was definitely a problem after GSK posted all the trials for the diabetes drug Avandia. A cardiologist from the Cleveland Clinic named Steve Nissan, accessed all of the reports and found that there was an excess of heart attacks on Avandia and not in the placebo in the same trial. This led to the perfect storm. What has become clear in the course of this is that an awful lot of the literature on Avandia was ghostwritten as well. What you find is that the FDA and the regulation in Europe, as well as the company ignored what should have been convincing data pointing to the fact that more people were having heart attacks on this drug than on placebo. They said the data are not statistically significant.

What you find is that the company reports a major trial that looked at the risks and gave the data to FDA, and the FDA in the first instance thought, well, as the company said, there is no big problem on this drug. It was only when one person in FDA dug through the material in greater detail that he found just this same kind of pattern that you see with the antidepressants. Hidden are the people who had had heart attacks and even died. They had been moved around. But the key way in which companies hides the data, and will always be able to hide the data unless things change, is the way that I am going to outline to you now. This may get a little bit more complicated, as you really have to be up early to keep up with the pharmaceutical companies. They now post all of their trials on the web, and the world thinks this is great. The *British Medical Journal* writes articles that this is a major new development and we should all feel much more relaxed in bed at night now. Well, what they are posting is study reports. They do not post the data. We have no more access to the data from these trials than we ever had before. They post study reports. The question is, which would you put more weight on, a company-authored study report or a ghostwritten article that academics have to agree to? I mean, it is not clear to me which of the two of those is the worst opposition.

The other thing is, when they post all of their trials, it is a little bit like trying to program a computer or the computer programming a man. You know, you have to make sure you know what the instructions are. You have to get the instructions just right or they don't do quite what you want. And the instructions to GSK of course are to hand over all of your clinical trials. Well, they don't. I mean, I have had a situation where GSK, as well as all of the companies have been asked, to hand over to FDA all of their clinical trials. They don't. So is GSK breaking the law? The answer is, no, they are not. GSK is, depending on the mood, a number of different companies. There is GSK central. And if GSK central is asked to hand over all their trials, they hand over all the trials that have begun in GSK central. But GSK France may not be exactly the same company, so they may not be legally obliged to hand over trials that had begun there, for instance. The other thing is, if they have got an inconvenient trial, they might go to Bob Whitaker, not a favored GSK person, and say, "Look, Bob. We need to run a trial on our drug" and say, "You know, here is what we think the protocol should be. Can you run this trial?"

Now it becomes Bob Whitaker's trial rather than GSK's trial. If it is likely to produce tricky results, it becomes Bob's trial rather than the company's trial. So when asked to hand over the Paxil trials, for instance, they will hand over ones that have been run by the company, but not Bob's.

The other thing is there is a bunch of coding terms. FDA had to be told the children who are emotionally labile on Paxil were actually suicidal. FDA did not know it. They did not look behind the data. They said, "Hey, a bunch of kids are just going emotionally labile on this drug. What's the problem?" So the key way to hide the data is to eliminate the patient. And this comes back to the empty stool that we have had earlier.

This is tricky, but two groups looking at the same data can come out with opposite observations. This is illustrated in the studies of Hommes, et al., and Missori, et al., in the use of subcutaneous heparin in the treatment of people who are at risk for DVTs. What you have got is two groups looking at subcutaneous heparin, and one group, Hommes et al., who say that subcutaneous heparin is the best way to treat people who are at risk for deep vein thrombosis. And you have a further group, Missori, et al., who says, no, these guys, Hommes, et al., they have got it all wrong. We have looked at the data too and we come to exactly the opposite conclusion to Hommes, et al. And Missori's letter gets published in the *Annals of Internal Medicine* (Missori, 1993), which is an extraordinarily good journal, and you are going to see this kind of disparity repeated again and again.

Looking at Figure 3, 95% is the confidence interval for this drug according to Missori, et al., the odd's ratio that it held was 0.61. But Hommes, et al., got an odd's ratio that the drug is going to be helpful on 0.62, almost precisely the same figure. But they have got a different confidence interval, and I am going to make it clear to you just why this is important.

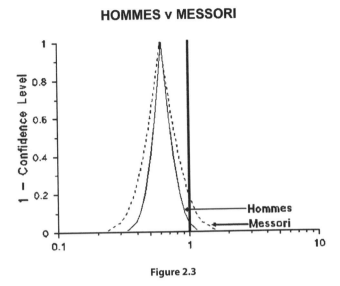

Figure 2.3

# What no effect looks like
RR=1.0

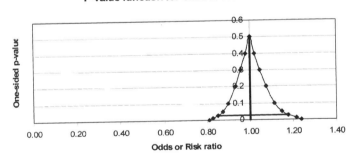

Figure 2.4

What is a confidence interval? Well, the data you have just seen comes from clinical trial material. We do clinical trials because the observations of doctors and therapists in tricky clinical situations are not reliable. We have a bias. We want to see the treatment working. The patient also wants to see the treatment working. So our observations are not terribly reliable in the case of tricky situations. If the patients are about to die from bacterial endocarditis and you give them penicillin and they get up off their deathbed and walk, your observations and the patient's observations that the drug probably made a difference are highly reliable. It is only when it is awfully tricky, when it is not clear that the treatment is all that good, but what you want to do is tease out to show it is working or not working enough, so that we need clinical trials and that your observations and mine may not be awfully reliable. So when we get the observations from a few hundred people together, you get a distribution of the results that looks like this. If the treatment is doing no good at all, the most common judgment we will have come to in a blind trial where we do not know what the actual treatment is and what the placebo is will be represented by the Figure 4. Okay? And then there will be a group review, who may have thought the treatment was helpful and your observations will be over on the left, and there will be a group of you who thought the treatment was unhelpful and your observations will be over here on the right. And your observations would be over here on the right if you thought it was unhelpful. Now, if Hommes and Missori have exactly the opposite results, you would expect Hommes, et al., to be over here on the left, completely, the whole curve to have moved there, and the Missori curve to be over on the right. That is what just the opposite results would look like. Okay? And what you get is, when you plot the data out from these two groups, you get two curves that look identical. These groups have produced almost exactly the same findings, but one group is saying that our observations are totally different to the other group. What is going on? I mean, this must look like double-Dutch to all of you. Well, you are in good company here, because anyone who knows a lot about statistics would agree with you. Okay? So you are feeling here, I don't understand this because I don't know much about statistics, when in actual fact, your instinctive judgments about what is going on here are exactly right. These results are identical. The point that is going on here is that this is the key to what the pharmaceutical companies do. Because the confidence interval crosses the line of 1.0 in Figure 3, this is the basis for Missouri, et al., saying that their results are totally different. This little bit of data here is the tail that is wagging the dog. Okay? Now, is this odd or unusual? And the answer is that far from being odd and unusual, it is the norm. Let me show you.

## Risk that Is Not Statistically Significant

When Prozac first got accused of causing people to commit suicide, there were a bunch of case reports from experienced therapists who had people come to them saying, "Doctor, I have been depressed before; I have been suicidal before. I've been put on this drug. This was something completely different to whatever happened to me before." Both the patient and the doctor produced observations that were very reliable. And when medical people or clinical people like you, looking at a patient having an adverse effect on a drug, say, "Well, look. I think this drug is doing this to the person right here in front of me." 80% of the time you are right. You have been told by the industry these days you are wrong, that we cannot depend on your judgment for these things, but actually 80% of the time you are right. An example is oral contraceptives and changes in your hair. Yes, oral contraceptives can change the quality of your hair. They can do all sorts of things to your hair. This was first reported in 1964 by patients reporting to doctors who then handed the reports on. These things are invariably right. However, what you have got was the company, Lily, saying, "Well, we have got all the clinical trial data. We have got hundreds of trials that have been done. We have meta-analyzed them and here they are in the *British Medical Journal*." Extrapolating to antidepressants, we are going to say, well, those anecdotes are over one-hundred. There are a few people talking about the fact that the patient has gone suicidal on the drug. The problem seems to clear up when you halt the drug and comes back when you go on the drug again, which should be cast iron proof the drug was causing a problem. What the companies do instead is to say, "We have taken all of our clinical trials and here they are, and what we can show is that the drug doesn't cause a problem."

However, when we take these data, what you find is that the rate of people who have gone on to a suicidal act on Prozac is increased. You see the curve. If there were no trouble while on the drug, the peak of the curve there, the red line, would coincide with the black line. That is 1.0 in Figure 4. If the drug were helping people so that you were less likely to become suicidal on Prozac than on placebo, the curve would be over on the left. But the curve is over on the right, saying that it is more likely you are going to go on to a suicidal act on Prozac. Okay? And it is roughly doubling of the risk. This is the risk that led FDA fifteen years later to put out a black box warning on the antidepressant. This is 1991. And this is adults, not children. And in the article in the *British Medical Journal*, what you have got is the company saying a thing that you and I can agree with, which is, when they look at the suicide acts on Prozac compared to placebo, that there is not a statistically significant difference between the two groups. There isn't. But what they go on to say, which you oughtn't to agree with and a 12-year-old child wouldn't have agreed with and people who know a lot about statistics wouldn't agree with, is that data from these trials do not show that the drug is associated with an increased risk. That is exactly wrong. The data show there is an increased risk. And this is the most common way for companies to hide problems, as I'm going to show you.

A hundred thousand people read the *British Medical Journal (BMJ)*. They are not all paid by the pharmaceutical industry. Most of them do not work in the mental health field. Lots of them aren't doctors. They are not making a living out of Prozac; they are not making a living out of drugs. None of them write in to the *BMJ* and say: Wait a minute here. There is an increased risk on this drug. So conflict-of-interest is not the problem. It is our problem in its own right, but it is not what is causing everything to go wrong. 1990 is the year that the first case reports come out saying that Prozac can be a problem. You will note, for three years beforehand, the clinical trial data showed there was an increased risk on this drug. FDA had hearings on the drug in 1991, where an awful lot of people went to the FDA to testify as part of the public. Women got up and talked about their husbands who had gone on to commit suicide, men who had often had the drug to help them stop smoking, and men who had had the drug to help them lose weight. They were not depressed. They had gone on this drug for a range of other reasons and a week or two later they had actually committed suicide. And what they were told was, "Well, these are all very sad stories, but your observations are unreliable. The reliable data show there is no problem." But, in fact, the reliable data show exactly the opposite. The reliable data were completely consistent with the observations of people who had loved ones who had committed suicide on this drug.

We talk about doctors being trained in evidence-based medicine these days and this is going to put the problem right. They have been trained to take exactly the view Lily took towards the data. If you take the opposite view and say, well, look, the data show that there is an increased risk; you are going to fail your medical exams these days. If the data are not statistically significant, then there is no increase in risk. Okay? And of course, if you are a company, it is awfully easy to make sure that the trials cannot become statistically significant, to engineer the trial, to make sure that the size of the trial means that the data will not ever become statistically significant. So you end up with the companies literally saying there is no evidence that our drug causes any problems at all. Let me show you this.

There are two other drugs that you will have heard about. First of all, Vioxx, which was used as a painkiller, and more recently Avandia, which has been used as a treatment for diabetes; in just the same way as with the SSRIs, what you got here was the companies publishing data. In the case of Vioxx, there was a big trial that had 4300 people on Vioxx and 4300 taking placebos. On the Vioxx, there were 17 heart attacks. On placebos, there were four. Now, there was a huge scandal when it later came out that Merck had hidden three dead bodies that were on Vioxx. There was an enormous scandal. In actual fact, they had hidden 14 dead bodies by saying, well, actually, 17 heart attacks on Vioxx is not statistically significant compared with four on placebo. They had to hide the three extra dead bodies, because, when you add those in, then 20 heart attacks become statistically significant. Do you see the issue? They can add or subtract any number of heart attacks in the trials. They can have a much greater number of heart attacks than reported. Are people going on to commit suicide? Are any other problems happening that are not statistically significant. Can they can depend on the doctor who will be treating them for respiratory problems, diabetes, or hypertension, to say, "You don't want to believe this, but this is no increase in risk." You may go, or you may have gone on Vioxx, and if you know the facts you may say, "Look, 17 heart attacks on Vioxx, 4 on placebo, you know doctor, I want off this drug." And your doctor is going to say to you there is no increase in risk. Not there. That is what you are up against. So let me show you a slightly different thing here.

## Who Is Most at Risk?

I have to give a talk next week in UCLA, and I was asked to declare conflicts-of-interest. Further, I have been told I have to put up a slide before the talk declaring what my conflicts-of-interest are. And this is what came to me, you know, I have got to actually disclose if I got any links to any of the pharmaceutical companies here, and what they would be happy with is that they want me to actually present material that is independent of industry-produced content. They only want material that is supported by published data and evidence-based guidelines.

Now I will put it to you that a person who has got links to Pfizer and Lily and GSK and who thinks that 17 heart attacks on Vioxx is a true increase compared with 4 on placebo is a much safer person to be talking to than a doctor who just goes by the guidelines. I may have jumped a little bit too quickly here. Industry controls all of the evidence that makes the guidelines. If you are a person going by the guidelines and have no links to any of the pharmaceutical companies, you are going to be much more in the pocket of industry than a person who has links to pharmaceutical companies. If I have got links to a pharmaceutical, as I have got links to almost all of them, you at least can see and know what you are dealing with and can scrutinize what I say. If I were a person who says I have got no links to the pharmaceutical industry, I am only going by the guidelines that are based on the published evidence; I am going to be much more in the pocket of the pharmaceutical industry than a person who has links to the industry. Further, I am going to be much more dangerous to you because I do not appear to have links. Do you see the problem?

There is a simple way to check this out if you want, if you are in clinical practice and want to know just what is going on. Drug A is a drug that is an antidepressant drug, or whatever, that can be helpful, maybe, but can also cause you to drop dead from whatever, maybe a heart attack. We have got good data on Drug A that shows there is a twofold increase in risk on Drug A of your getting a heart attack, and this is statistically significant. And then you have got Drug B, on which we have got loads of data on it as well. There is roughly an eightfold increase in risk, but, in fact, the data are not statistically significant. And the question is:

Which drug should you take? Now, most of you here in the room probably will come to the right answer quite quickly, which is that Drug B is four times more risky than Drug A. The one you do not want to be on is Drug B. What the pharmaceutical industry is in the business of trying to say to you is that Drug A is the risky drug. Because the data on Drug B is not statistically significant, you do not need to worry about the problem. The situation is a bit like this: In the case of Drug A, you have got a gun that has six barrels to it and you know for sure there is one bullet in one of the barrels. In the case of Drug B, you had a quick glimpse of the barrel as it has been spun, and you got the impression that there are bullets in there, but you are not absolutely sure what is going on. Maybe it is just that the barrel was spun too quickly. In fact, there are three or four bullets in there, but you do not know that for sure. The industry is trying to say to you, because you do not know for sure that there are no bullets in there that the only safe gun to play Russian roulette with is the one that has the confirmed bullet in one barrel. That is the situation you are in, we are all in, as regards healthcare, not just for the antidepressant, but for Lipitor, asthma drugs, any kind of drugs that you care to think of.

## The Industry's View

This hopefully brings us back to the child-abuse issue beautifully, which is the industry view of things. If FDA were to send out information that there seems to be an increased risk of people becoming suicidal on Prozac based on data that is not statistically significant or increased risk of heart attacks on Vioxx based on the data there are 17 heart attacks on Vioxx compared to 4 on placebo, that this is just a signal. And that is a bit as if your neighbor said to you that, well; I think you're a pedophile. Now, at the end of the day it was proven that you are not a pedophile, and you end up having been proven right, but by then your reputation has been trashed. The industry is saying, well, look, it is not fair to trash our reputation; it is not fair to trash the drug until you have proved beyond doubt that the drug causes a problem. Right? And of course, as I said to you, the industry runs the trials and they can make sure that the data never becomes statistically significant. It is quite like the Catholic Church operating a Canon Law system. You know, they do not operate by the laws of the U.S. or European Union, or whatever. They have got Canon Law. They have got their own legal system, and according to this, well, the priests are not ever actually proven to be guilty.

There is a case as it stands today in front of the Supreme Court in the U.S. where the pharmaceutical industry is arguing just that unless the data are statistically significant, we do not need to put it in the label of the drug. Okay? There is a bunch of judges who have been asked to see if they actually agree with this or not, judges who hold stakes in pharmaceutical companies, who are being asked, well, you know, do you want the companies that you hold shares in to have to put in the label of the drug adverse effects of this drug on the basis of pretty convincing data the drug does cause a problem, but state that it is not statistically significant?

On the other hand, you have Raptiva, which has been withdrawn from the market on the basis of three patients developing a condition that I have actually forgotten the name. It is some extraordinary large medical condition, something like polymononuclear leukodystrophy or whatever. Three patients had the problem and the FDA withdrew the drug immediately. What we are living in is a world where it can be very clear that your observations or the patient's observations are absolutely right and you need to upgrade on the basis of that, and what I'm keen to do is try and work out how we can get back to a world where your observations count as there's a world where the industry seems to be able to say that your observations don't count. And that's what we need to counter. You have never seen a controlled trial of a parachute. If you did, all of the dead bodies would be over on the right in which they had a placebo instead of a parachute and all of the live bodies would be on the left. You have never seen a controlled trial of an antibiotic for bacterial endocarditis because, if you did, most of the dead bodies would be in the untreated group and most of the living people would be in the treated group. Not everybody that got the drug would live, not everybody who got the placebo would die, but the data would look like something in that direction.

In the United Kingdom, we have universal healthcare. It's not on the basis that we have been touchy-feely 50 years ago and thought it was a nice thing to do. It seemed to be a good investment to give free healthcare with drugs like the antibiotics to people who are at risk of dying or people who are going to be out of work and disabled, because with drugs like these, you got people up off their deathbed and you put them back to work and it meant that we were better able to compete with Germany and France and places like that. It was an investment. But it is different in the case of drugs like the statins and potentially drugs like the antidepressants and all sorts of other drugs that don't save lives, and where in the clinical trials of these drugs you have got more people dying on the active drug than on the placebo, and with which we are getting all sorts of adverse effects from the drugs and becoming neurotic because of the side effects of their drugs. In that case, you have got the kinds of situations where universal healthcare is potentially a disaster. Potentially, we in the U.K. are in big, big trouble if we make available for free statins and the antidepressants and a range of other drugs like this, because what you've got here is an expense rather than an investment.

This is what the data on the antidepressants looks like, and this is from the FDA and not me. When they asked for all of the trials, what they got were one-hundred-thousand people on placebo-controlled trials. When they looked at the data, the antidepressants beat the placebo marginally. But this is a rating scale beating. There are more dead bodies in the drug column than in the placebo column. It depends on your choice of outcome measure. You can say that the antidepressants work, or you can say, well actually, if the issue is trying to keep people alive or get people back to work, there is literally no evidence that the antidepressants work at all. That's not saying they can't be helpful. I think they can be helpful. The issue is what's going on in controlled trials and what has the industry been able to do? Controlled trials began as a way to screen out snake oil, to show that drugs didn't work. What they have become on the basis of data like this, they have become the fuel for therapeutic bandwagons, which is not what they were supposed to be. Industry, on the basis of data like this, says the drug has been shown to work; therefore, you must get it. When, in actual fact, if you are going to be evidence-based, you could argue that, well, 80% of the response to the drug that you have just seen in Figure 3 stems from nonspecific or placebo factors. So if you are going to be evidence-based, you would wait. When the patient comes in to you first, you would wait. You wouldn't jump into an antidepressant. You would look at lifestyle issues, behavioral issues, you'd say to the patient that the natural history of the condition you have is that it's going to potentially clear up in a few weeks anyway if you just wait, and I'll wait with you. And if that fails, then you have antidepressants to turn to or antipsychotics or whatever. But we are not actually following what the data show. We're following what industry portrays the data as showing.

As I said to you, one of the other issues to bear in mind with the antidepressant drugs or the antipsychotic drugs, we don't have good evidence of people getting back to work or remaining alive. We have got changes on a rating scale. In the case of the antidepressant trials, it's mainly the Hamilton Rating Scale for Depression. In almost all the trials of the SSRIs, they used quality-of-life scales as well that were filled by the patient, which rated issues that were of more interest to the patient. And there have been over a hundred trials in which these scales were used and the data remains universally unpublished because, when the patients did the rating, the drug didn't work at all. Rating scales would be a reasonable way to look at the outcomes if across all of these domains of measurement we got the same answer, the drug beats placebo. We don't. It's only in this domain here that we get the answer that the drug appears to work. And industry again is able, along with academia, to run with this, saying that we've got a change in just this one area here and that trumps everything else.

One final point, as we're in the denouement. Of all the people that respond to antidepressants, there is only one, essentially, out of ten who is showing a specific response to the drug. Even though four out of ten show a response, it's to placebo or nonspecific factors. And then there's a further group of people who show no good response at all. So that's nine people out of ten. Now, if I put you on an antidepressant and if something strange happens to you, such as you turn blue and grow feathers, what happens? If I write to the *BMJ* and say that I put Nick on an antidepressant, he turned blue, and grew feathers, and when we stopped the drug, he turned back to a good shade, a normal pink shade, the *BMJ* will say that's just an anecdote. We don't take reports like this anymore. We only take controlled trials.

In actual fact, what we've really got here is the *BMJ* taking a new form of anecdote. They're taking material that privileges the experience of this one person here and discounts the experience of these nine here. This is not good science. So how do we solve the problem?

## Can Doctors Solve the Problem?

Well, there are two ways to solve the problem. There are two approaches. And I'm going to give you the standard approach towards trying to solve the problem; this is a top-down approach.

This says sit back, relax, don't bother your little heads; the experts are going to sort it out for you. That's what we have experts for. Okay? That's a shower approach. The other approach is the bidet approach, from the bottom up. Okay? And as you will see, this is the one that I think we should opt for. I intended to take a vote and see which of you favor the shower approach and which of you favor the bidet approach, but now that you've been told that the bidet approach is one that I favor—and Stockholm syndrome means you're only going to get out of this room if you agree with me—you will all vote for the bidet approach, so the vote has been canceled.

What is the shower approach? Well, doctors care, and we all agree they do, they do care. But they're trapped. They're as much trapped as the patient is. We could argue, and we should argue, you don't want to completely ignore the shower approach, but what we've got is evidence-based medicine for the moment. You're told, if only we practiced evidence-based medicine, everything will be okay. Everybody assumes that means data-based medicine, and that's the problem: It doesn't. The data are hidden. The company has the trials. They have produced the bits of the data that suit them. You don't get access to all of the data. We should be insisting on access to all of the data. If I got up here and said to you, I have a treatment that works for whatever and you ask to see the data and I refused to show it to you, I would be run out of town. But the industry does this the whole time. They get up and they present the evidence and I or you ask for the data, and they say, "Get lost. No one sees the data." The regulators don't see it. In essence, nobody does. Okay? So what we need is: we need to replace evidence-based medicine with data-based medicine. You've seen in industry that for their points of view, they use statistical models also to hide the data. Unless it's statistically significant, it's not the data that counts. We need to get back to a world in which the increased number of heart attacks, even if it's not statistically significant, counts. We can say to the government that it's just not working, but that poses the government a big problem, which is, well, if we're going to solve the problem, the only rational way forward is evidence-based medicine. If you're not going to practice evidence-based medicine, you're being irrational. So we have got to find another way forward. We can say to the government that you'd save money, that newer, poorer, inferior drugs are pushing out older, better treatments generally. And that so far hasn't worked. And I have been intrigued with some of the health providers here in the States. I'm from Europe, a softy kind of place. You've got a rough, tough market economy here. I'm always intrigued by the health insurers and health providers, and I don't understand why they don't get to grips with this. They could say, "Look, we've been asked to pay through the nose for treatments that are much more expensive that aren't working and we're going to refuse. We want good data and we're going to go by that." But the insurers and providers and all seem to be trapped in the same way.

What the problem is if you're going to take a shower approach, for most doctors and experts, the problem is a little bit like the ski run in Mammoth, not too far away from here. This is the Paranoids run to those of you who have been to Mammoth. You've got a bunch of what looks like fairly tough hombres up at the top. Even they are saying, how am I supposed to go down this? And that's what the problem has become for a lot of doctors who mean well. Can I survive going over the edge of this, saying that evidence-based medicine is really not the right way forward. Even just to say that sounds wrong.

One of the answers people have come up with is, well, let's force industry to do comparative effectiveness research by comparing different forms of treatment. If we get them to show the one, such as let's say the older treatment turns out to be superior to the new treatment, then, we won't reimburse the new treatment, this will put things right. It won't.

Let me explain the situation I think we're in. Imagine a situation where you broke an arm and you went in to your local ER and they said, "Good news. We're running a controlled trial in here of treatments for broken arms, and what we're going to do is: we are going to randomize you if you're happy." And of course you'll say you're happy because you know you have to keep the doctor happy or you're not going to get out with your arm fixed. "We're going to randomize you to either no plaster cast or a plaster cast on your right arm or your left arm or your right leg or your left leg even though you've broken your right arm. Okay?" Now, the data from that kind of trial would show that plaster casts beat placebo, even though in only one in four cases it's been put on the right arm. That's all it will take for the plaster cast to beat placebo. And out of that you get the recommendation: Put a plaster cast on some limb and it's going to be better than placebo. It's a recipe for not thinking. Comparative effectiveness research just says, well, when the patient comes in, put two plaster casts on, one on the right leg and one on the left arm, even though they've broken the right arm. And if you do a trial like that, you will show that two plaster casts randomly applied will beat one. If that's the kind of data that control the healthcare you give, it's unthinking. It isn't the way forward. Of course, if you take it to its logical conclusion, you'll say, we will beat placebo by the greatest amount if we put the patient in a full-body plaster cast. This will always beat the placebo. But that's all we've been asked to do when we have been asked to go by data like this without thinking about what the underlying problem is.

Now we're back to the Church and we're back to the issue of doctors in particular and maybe all of us in healthcare. Do we still have the credibility that's needed to put the problem right? Do you think doctors at the moment are any more inclined than the Cardinals in the U.S. have been to put the problem right?

Putting it in a slightly different way will answer it. Do you think doctors are a revolutionary class? Well, if you watch

*House* on TV you may even recall from an episode from season four, I think the fourth episode. Foreman had left and had gone to a different hospital, but was applying the approach he had learned from House. He had a very tricky case where he did all the orthodox health-care things and the patient seemed to be getting worse, and in the end he did an unorthodox thing and saved the person's life. The episode ends, of course, with the administrator from the hospital saying, well, that was great medicine, but bad healthcare, so you're sacked. Now, that was fictional but, and I hope I'm not stealing Bob's thunder too much, that's happening today again and again and again. There's an article from Israel about a controlled trial where what they did was to remove patients from the drugs they were on. These were older patients and they systematically reduced the number of drugs these people were on. They were able to show, in essence, that reducing the number of drugs drastically reduced the number of dead bodies. Those that were on less drugs were less likely to die. Just to repeat the point: These were not mental healthcare drugs. These were drugs across medicine. This is not just a mental healthcare issue. This is a healthcare issue. You reduce the number of drugs, you were less likely to die, less likely to go into hospital, less likely to have adverse events of any sort.

There's good evidence for reducing polypharmacy that it will be helpful. Why do we have polypharmacy? We've got polypharmacy because we have got guidelines for diseases. We don't have guidelines for people. If you had a guideline for people, one of the things it would say is that polypharmacy is a bad thing. Polypharmacy is a disorder that needs to be treated, and you go about treating it by reducing the number of drugs.

The situation we're in is a little bit is like an instance in the United Kingdom recently where there was consternation in an area of the U.K. called the Lake District. This area has small little roads and stone walls and things like that, but there were these huge juggernaut trucks roaring off the motorway, down these lanes, knocking over the walls and houses and getting stuck in small little towns. Everybody was angry with all this and wondered how it had happened. And it had happened because the guys with the trucks were using GPS. They had a device that said there's a delay up ahead, turn off onto this road, which they did. And that's what's happening in medicine these days. Doctors and everyone else in healthcare aren't driving by their instincts, by what they see in front of them. They're not using common sense. The guideline says, "turn off." The guideline says, for diabetes add this drug, for hypertension add this, for depression add this, so people end up on fifteen different drugs. Nothing is there saying this does not make sense to have people on this number of drugs.

Mark Foster, whom Bob knows, and whom you can read, may be able to tell you more. He outlined how he tried to get people off drugs. It's a dangerous thing to pay heed to people like Bob. Mark did. And he tried to get the people that came to see him off the different drugs they were on. He showed extremely beneficial outcomes, and this week, a few days ago; the boss walked in and said, "You're sacked. You're not keeping to the standard of care."

So what would the bidet approach look like? You would want a patient reporting adverse events. There are a few things you can do. You can explain to patients, I've got a drug that's been shown in ten people to be helpful. I mean, all it took was ten people for this drug to be shown to be helpful, and now I've got a drug that was in a controlled trial where ten thousand people were recruited to the trial. Which would you prefer to have? Well, the doctor would prefer you to have the drug that was in the trial that involved ten thousand people, and you would, too. This would sound good. Whereas, in actual fact, you put snake oil into a trial with one-hundred or two-hundred people or maybe one thousand people and it can be shown to work. Recruiting thousands of people to a trial is a recipe for showing ineffective treatments have a marginal effect. You want to explain to patients quite easily, you really only want to be on drugs where extremely few people need to be recruited to the trial to show that it works. It's the example of a parachute. You know, any N=1 is all it takes when a treatment really works. But aside from that, if you look at what industry does, they track every single script a doctor writes. This is good business. Doctors, in contrast, if anyone has an adverse effect on a drug, if you get killed by the drug, they only report one in a hundred of the adverse effects have happened to you. These things go in to the FDA who regards them as anecdotes and does nothing about them. If they go to the company, it says there is a bunch of people over in Phoenix who are saying people turn blue on Prozac. We're going to send the company people out to Phoenix in particular to show how the clinical trials don't show that Prozac turns you blue. You know, we've got a job to do here in Phoenix. The answer to the problem I think is to give a megaphone back to the patient and potentially to the prescriber also. If it is a doctor, it's more likely that a clinical psychologist would be open to this. Others within the healthcare system who have prescribing privileges can also help the patient. And the idea would be this: to get a patient to report to a website about an adverse effect on a drug. The doctor, if they happen to report that you had a problem on a drug like lithium or a bunch of heart drugs that can cause you to have what doctors report as ataxia, they will report just that one word to FDA, ataxia. If you give patients the opportunity to report, they more likely will report, I became dis-coordinated on the drug. The first time it happened, I fell down the stairs and broke my leg and ended up in hospital. The most recent time it happened, I was driving the car and I crashed and can't drive anymore while I'm on this drug and I have now lost my job. You see the economic impact of this can be enormous. When in fact, we're paying more on treating the adverse effects of drugs these days than we are on the entire drug's budget. You hear the drug's budget is crippling us.

It's not. It's treating the adverse effects of drugs that's crippling us at the moment.

Well, what we need to do is, I think, get patients to report because doctors don't. They're causing a Stockholm syndrome-type situation. They don't report to the doctor straight and then get the doctor to report on. You've got to get them to report, maybe with your help. They should then, I think, from a website get a letter that prints out the report in which they've given the problem, and what the evidence is that other people have had this kind of problem. A letter that they can take back to the doctor, saying nice things to the doctor, like 80% of the time your observations are likely to be right. You know, 80% of the time the patients' observations are likely to be right as well. We just say to the doctor, 80% of the time his or her observations are likely to be right, compared with the clinical trial data that he's relying on which is not reliable. The idea is to get the doctor to also report, with feedback on the basis of both reports to the patient and the doctor that, well, there's a thousand of you who reported this particular problem on the drug and there's a hundred doctors or clinical psychologists or maybe pharmacists who have endorsed in their opinion that there is a link.

What I'm trying to do is to reverse the Stockholm syndrome here, to reverse the isolation that both patients and clinical psychologists, doctors, social workers, and others are in at the moment. I think as therapists and patients, we're in a profoundly isolated situation. It's increasingly clear to me and also to other people who are in our work where, if I don't keep to what the guidelines say, I'm going to lose my job, which is close to death in its own right. Okay. So it's a tricky situation for both doctors and patients.

This is the bind that we're caught in. This is the way I think. I mean, I think we need a bidet approach. What I'm doing here is asking you a question: How do we bring that kind of thing into being? How do we make it scientifically respectable? So, thank you.

# References

Cipriani, A., Furukawa, T.A., Salanti, G., et al. (2009). Comparative efficacy and acceptability of 12 new-generation antidepressants: A multiple-treatments meta-analysis. *Lancet,* 373, 746-758.

Keller, M.B., Ryan, N.D., Strober, M., et al. (2001). Efficacy of in the treatment of adolescent major depression: A randomized, controlled trial. *Child and Adolescent Psychiatry,* 40(7), 762-772.

Messori, L., et al (1993). A meta-analysis of six randomized trials comparing subcutaneous heparin with continuous intravenous heparin for the treatment of deep vein thrombosis. *Annals of Internal Medicine,* 118, 77-78.

Chapter 3

# Patient Bill of Rights for Psychotropic Medication

*(Edited from the transcription of the presentation)*

*David Antonuccio, Ph.D.*

W ell, it's a pleasure to be here. I've really enjoyed the presentations so far, and I am going to try to build on the concept of the bottom-up approach with what I'm referring to as a Patient Bill of Rights for Psychotropic Medication. The Bill of Rights is the name of the first ten amendments to the U.S. Constitution introduced by James Madison to the First U.S. Congress in 1789. The Bill of Rights limits the power of the U.S. Federal Government, protecting the natural rights of liberty and property, including freedom of speech, free press, free assembly, free association, and the right to keep and bear arms, as well as speed in public trial with an impartial jury, freedom from cruel and unusual punishment, and freedom from criminal double jeopardy. Dr. Barry Duncan and I have put together what we are calling and proposing as a Bill of Rights designed to preserve the autonomy and freedom of patients who are prescribed psychotropic drugs, and so this is an evolving document, and there may be ideas that you have for how to make it better. And I can tell you that both Dr. Duncan and I are open to those, and we want to make it a document that will grow and get better in time. So here we go.

# Right Number One

The first principle is: Patients have a right to a thorough diagnostic and functional assessment by a behavioral health-care specialist. Patients with mental health issues need a thorough physical examination and treatment by providers who understand the connection between medical and psychological health. This usually involves a team approach, and psychologists are uniquely qualified as behavioral scientists to be part of that team. And often there are medical disorders that go undetected or undiagnosed and masquerade as psychiatric conditions. This is from a study done a few years ago (Koran et al., 2002) where they looked at consecutive admissions for psychiatric patients at a public psychiatric hospital, and 29% had a medical disorder, 8% had a newly diagnosed medical disorder, and almost 6% had a medical disorder that may have caused or exacerbated their psychiatric disorder. So it's important for patients who present with psychiatric problems to have a thorough physical examination to rule out some sort of undiagnosed medical condition. So the link between the medical and the psychological is very important.

But, also, substances can play a role. This was a study done at one of the Southern California V.A. Hospitals by Brown and Schuckit (1988) a number of years ago, and they looked at veterans who were drinking every day, and 42% of them had clinically significant levels of depression. But when they stopped drinking for four weeks, this dropped down to only 6%. So sometimes the symptoms that you're seeing are being caused by, or at least exacerbated, by some other drug or medication, and it's important to recognize that, and providers need to be aware of that.

There are a number of different prescription drugs that can cause depression, and it's important to know about those as well. So everything is linked, and as psychologists we need to know about these links in order to properly help our patients.

## Right Number Two

Patients have a right to be informed about the safety and efficacy of treatment options, including psychological treatment alone, medication alone, psychological treatment combined with medication, as well as what the outcome would be if they did not receive any treatment at all. So informing patients about side effects is important. Lots of people don't know what can happen when you combine various drugs, and a lot of people don't know that taking antidepressants are the most common agents used in suicide by poisoning. They are involved in over half of the serious adult overdoses. SSRIs appear to have the same risk of overdose as tricyclic antidepressants, although in theory they are less deadly when used alone, but they are often not prescribed alone or used alone. Antidepressants are prescribed with other psychotropic drugs over half the time. So it's very, very common. There was a Canadian study in 2001 that showed that SSRI-related deaths are most likely to occur when patients take two or more other drugs, including alcohol, in conjunction with them. In a study done in Massachusetts of Medicaid patients, 5000 patients were on two or more antidepressants, more than 1100 patients were on five, six, or seven different psychotropic drugs at a time. So this is a practice that is common particularly in the poor, and it's something that is dangerous. And, again we are usually as a psychologist reluctant to say anything about it, but we need to start saying something about it, and we need to educate our patients so they can do something about it themselves.

# Right Number Three

Patients have a right to be informed that there is no evidence of a chemical imbalance causing any mental disorder, nor is there any evidence that psychotropic drugs fix a chemical imbalance. Of course this goes contrary to the marketing of most of the psychotropic drugs that are used out there, and a lot of times when people see this, they can hardly believe it. If you were to do a survey and ask how many people think depression is caused by a chemical imbalance that's been identified in the scientific literature, probably most would say that's the case. But it's not true.

We are unlikely to isolate a depression gene, as most disorders have input from multiple genes, and also their expression is related to environmental influences. Yet we definitely tend to think of these conditions as medical diseases, but the DSM does not even specify, to get the disorder, that there has to be an identified medical condition, and they say these disorders don't represent disease entities per se. But that is certainly not how we operate in this world. We see them as medical diseases requiring medical intervention. I'll read to you this caption. It says: "You're not the only person in the world who's depressed. You're the only person in the world who's not taking antidepressants." And there's no doubt antidepressants have become very popular, yet the efficacy data do not warrant their popularity. The stuff that Dr. Healy presented shows that they are just marginally more effective than placebo. And of course the risk data, when you consider that, then you really start to wonder if the risk-benefit analysis leads to a conclusion that they're more effective and safe, and I'm not sure they are.

Antidepressant use has grown tremendously. As of 2004, the revenue estimates for antidepressants topped $13 billion annually. The revenues for SSRIs have been growing about 25% each year. Some estimates suggest that one in eight adult Americans has taken an antidepressant in the prior ten years. Of those taking antidepressants, about 60% indicate they have taken them for more than three months. 46% have taken them for more than a year. This is so despite the fact that most antidepressant trials last only six weeks. So we're often in uncharted territory in terms of the longer-term use, which tends to be the case, at least in our culture. In fact, Prozac and other SSRIs have taken on mythical powers: [read from cartoon] "Of course your daddy loves you. He's on Prozac. He loves everybody." They are seen as powerful, even life-saving and transforming, and it's transfused into cartoons. These cartoons reflect the cultural belief that this is what happens when you take these drugs, despite what the data show.

The scientific literature gives us an idea of how effective these antidepressants versus placebo generally are. Irving Kirsch, a colleague of ours, has done wonderful meta-analyses that have received worldwide acclaim, deservedly so (Kirsch, 2010). But, basically, the average placebo patient does 82% as well as the average active drug patient. In other words, the placebo duplicates 82% of the effects that you see with the active drug. Further, there is some question about whether that extra benefit, that marginal benefit, attributed to the drug is really a true drug effect or some kind of enhanced placebo due to the side effects that undoubtedly un-blind these studies.

And of course benefit is only half the story. Risk is important, and it is the providers who are supposed to weigh benefit and risk, both. And the FDA analysis of all the antidepressant trials showed the active drug basically doubled the risk of serious suicide-related events compared to placebo.

Now this translates to about 4% of the patients on the active drug becoming suicidal versus 2% on the placebo. So there are two extra suicidal patients for every hundred treated with the antidepressant. Okay. And the way I refer to this is this way: that the risk is low, but the stakes are high. If it happens to be you or your family member who is among those extra two, it's quite serious.

An FDA analysis of all antidepressant trials for both SSRIs and SNRIs in regard to suicide-related events (N=4250) reveals that such untoward events are 2:1 higher with antidepressants. This is why so many of these medications have a black-box warning.

I want to present a little bit of data from what I consider one of the best comparative studies ever done on depression, and this happens to be The Treatment of Adolescent Depression Study (TADS, 2004). The lead author is John March, but a lot of wonderful scientists are involved in the study. It has provided as much data on risk as it did on efficacy, which differs from most studies that sort of highlight the efficacy and ignore the risk data. So this study allowed you to put the data in a graph so a reader could go through and look at the increased risks associated with the medications. This was published in the *Journal of the American Medical Association (JAMA)* in an exceptionally well designed, executed, and well-written study. These are the results that were highlighted in the media, and shown here in Figure 1. Basically you have got four conditions: (a) combined condition, (b) Fluoxetine or Prozac alone, (c) CBT alone, and (d) placebo treatment. The patients were randomly assigned to 12 weeks of treatment. This study shows that on one measure, the Clinicians Global Index (CGI) that the combined condition had the best outcome. And, you know, the way I see it: Live by the data, die by the data. CBT did not do as well in this study as hoped, at least on this measure, but it's important to note that the CGI is the clinicians' rating for global improvement. This is not the primary depression measure. When you look at the primary depression measure, the placebo duplicated 86% of the drug in this study on something called the Children's Depression Research Scale, and this was not statistically significant. This, again, is the typical relationship you will see between placebo and the active drug. The FDA did not count this study as a positive study for Fluoxetine because of this result. And it should be noted, also, that CBT did not separate from the placebo statistically. So, you know, placebo does pretty well in these studies, and some people see that as a negative. But what I think it means is that the psychological benefits of a therapeutic alliance and a focus on problem-solving, along with confidentiality and other of these nonspecific effects are powerful and they should not be minimized. We ought not to apologize for them. They may be a critical ingredient to what makes psychotherapy effective as well.

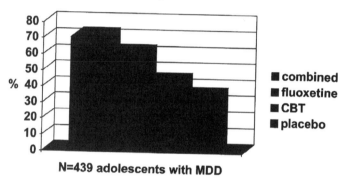

## TADS Study (2004)
### Acute Response on CGI

N=439 adolescents with MDD

combined
fluoxetine
CBT
placebo

Figure 3.1

But, again, we don't want to just look at benefit. We want also to look at harm. Those patients who received Fluoxetine were twice as likely to have a harm-related adverse event, and this was the same relationship that was uncovered in the FDA analysis that combined all the antidepressant studies. That is why Prozac also has the black-box warnings. This difference was statistically signifi-cant. And it's worth noting that suicidality decreased across all four conditions in this study. Here we've got the two Fluoxetine condi-tions combined and two non-Fluoxetine conditions combined. But it decreased in all four conditions, so this is a relative risk that we're seeing. And, also, keep in mind, that this study, along with most antidepressant studies, excluded suicidal patients before the study was even started. In other words, they could not get into the study in the first place. And so you have a low base rate to start with, but still this relationship emerged. So these are the results for Prozac, the only FDA-approved drug for depression in kids.

Figure 2 shows the non-psychiatric adverse events from the Treatment of Adolescence Study (TADS, 2004). These are all the non-psychiatric adverse events that had an odds ratio of greater than 2, and that is the drug condition was more than twice as likely to cause this particular side effect compared to placebo: sedation, GI problems, diarrhea, flu, insomnia, sinus problem, and vomiting. Okay?

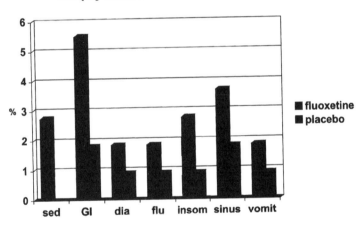

Figure 3.2

So, again, if you do what is conventionally done and just pay attention to benefits and completely ignore side effects and harm-related events and adverse events, you will come to different conclusions for what is the best treatment.

In 2007, there was a thirty six week follow-up data for the three primary conditions only (combined, CBT, and Fluoxetine) because it did not continue the placebo condition, and there were no statistically significant differences. On the basis of the TADS study, the authors concluded that, "The medical management of major depressive disorder with Fluoxetine, including careful monitoring for adverse events, should be made widely available, not discouraged."

My colleague David Burns and I took exception to that conclusion because we felt the conclusions ignored the harm data that were clearly present in the study, and so we wrote a response to that in *JAMA* that was published, figuring that what's important is balancing benefit and risk. Again, the follow-up data at 36 weeks, showed no significant differences. Further, a five-year follow-up study was recently published that also found no significant differences among the three groups. It is interesting, that overall, 96% of these kids recovered from their index episode, while 47% had a recurrence. In this, recurrence is fairly common, but most of these kids ended up recovering from the episode with clinical treatment. But, again, weighing the risk data at the follow-up, and looking at just suicidal events, CBT had the lowest rate, followed by the combination condition, and then the Fluoxetine alone had the highest rate of suicidal events. This all has to be factored into the patients' decision tree about whether or not to use a particular treatment, in this case the parents' decision tree about whether to use it for their depressed child.

## Right Number Four

Another right, we think, is that patients have a right to be treated with psychosocial interventions alone if they so choose. Maybe not so much anymore, but this has been something that would raise eyebrows in years past when I would say something like this because the assumption is, well, if someone is really depressed, you got to get them on the drugs, don't you? And fortunately, for depression, anyway, that's not the case. The psychological treatments do as well alone as a standalone treatment, and even in the case of severe depression, fortunately there are a number of psychological options available to us as therapists. There is cognitive therapy, as well as the emphasizing of modified expectations. This is the era of reduced expectations: [read from cartoon] "Well, if everything goes okay that old left foot should be coming into view soon." And sometimes with patients, you almost have to lower the bar this low to help them set goals with which they can have successful experiences and build on those.

We're also trying to teach people not to be so hard on themselves: [read from cartoon] "While extortion, racketeering, and murder may be bad acts, they don't make you a bad person." I don't have time to present you all of the data on cognitive therapy, so I'm going to list just a few examples, but there's a lot of scientific data supporting it.

- Couples counseling
- Exposure therapy for anxiety
- Mindfulness therapy, helping people balance their lives
- Behavioral activation, getting people moving again

The key is, finding that elusive balance as professionals, and it's hard for professionals to do that, and sometimes what we think is successful can be also stressful. Positive changes, promotions, that sort of thing, buying a house, all of that, all the trappings of success can also be stressful and get you out of balance.

The general assumption out there is that if you're severely depressed, you really need to get on antidepressants, and we're afraid to challenge that usually. So what I've tried to do over the course of my career is write articles that summarize the data to arm the clinician, researcher clinician, scientist, to say, well, that's not true. These data show that it's not.

DeRubeis (2005) and Steve Hollon (Holon et al., 2005) are probably the two greatest depression researchers of our era. They're kind of like the Rolling Stones or something, as far as I'm concerned, just real rock stars. And they have done some of the best studies I've ever seen. And this was one that looked at the most severely depressed patients. They selectively recruited and enrolled moderate-to-severely depressed patients by any criteria. They had to have a score of 20 or more on the Modified Seventeen-Item Hamilton Scale. So anyway, they had to carry a diagnosis of major depression. The patients were randomly assigned to sixteen weeks of cognitive therapy, sixteen weeks of medication, or eight weeks of pill placebo medication. The medication was Paxil, up to 50 mg daily, augmented by lithium or Desipramine if necessary. There were two-hundred forty patients enrolled in this study. It was published in the *Archives of General Psychiatry*. Response was defined as a Hamilton score of twelve or lower. So at eight weeks, the active treatments were doing better than the placebo, so they, for ethical reasons, decided to stop the placebo condition. And then at sixteen weeks, you can see visually that the medication and the cognitive therapy had the same response rate. Okay? Again, response is important. But we also want to know about sustained improvement. They continued treatment of responders from the study for one more year with the responders. There were one-hundred four responders and this was the outcome at the end of that. Of the patients who had sustained improvement (i.e., did not have any relapse at all) those that got cognitive therapy plus three booster sessions had the best outcome. Those in the antidepressant condition prior were randomly assigned to either continue on pill placebo for a year or antidepressant for a year, and those that continued on the antidepressant did somewhat better than those that were switched to pill placebo. But the cognitive therapy group with the booster sessions had the best outcome.

Of the remitted patients at the end of the acute phase, and looking at the percentage of patients that relapsed, those withdrawn from cognitive therapy were less likely to relapse than those who were withdrawn from medications. Those continuing on antidepressants did not have as good an outcome (i.e., more likely to relapse) as those just given the cognitive therapy with a few booster sessions.

Again, these are severely depressed patients by any measure. So these data should put a stake in the heart of the myth that if someone is really severely depressed, they have to have the antidepressants.

Then what they did was to take forty patients who remained active and did not relapse during the continuation phase and followed them for another year with no treatment intervention at all. These patients who had had prior cognitive therapy were much less likely to relapse. There are many studies that show this, as did this study, that the patients were learning some skills to prevent relapse. You know, the old saying, you can give a hungry man fish and feed him for a day or teach him how to fish and feed him for a lifetime, and the idea here is to teach the skills that will help the person cut short or prevent future episodes of depression.

## Rights Number Five

Patients have a right to be exposed to the fewest side effects and the low risk of adverse events from psychotropic medications, a right to a first-do-no-harm approach. And part of the idea behind this Bill of Rights is that patients will be empowered, and with their Bill of Rights in hand, can go to their doctors and say, "I want to see a doctor that prescribes according to these principles," because teaching the doctors doesn't seem to be working. Relying on the scientific journals, as Dr. Healy pointed out, doesn't seem to be working, so we, I think, need to empower the patients to demand the kind of treatment that we think is both safe, effective, and ethical. Along with this principle, probably there should be a corollary, which would be something like: Combining medications in the absence of evidence should be something that is not done. Yet, as we know, it's actually fairly common. And of course you run the risk of what's called a prescribing cascade: [reads from cartoon] "The problem is, you're overmedicated. Luckily there are drugs that can help you with that."

The side effects and risks of medication combinations are often unknown or underappreciated. One of my graduate students and I did a review in which we were looking for antidepressant augmentation studies. The meta-analysis found that the combination was not significantly better than the mono therapy. And of course there are going to be many more risks. About 80% of patients experience side effects from antidepressants as mono therapies. Common side effects of the SSRIs include agitation, sleep disruption, sexual dysfunction, and gastrointestinal problems. And I have been contending that part of the problem with these antidepressants is that they are called antidepressants in the first place. They could just as easily be called, you know, erection impairment drugs, you know, agitation enhancers, or something like that, but they're not likely to sell as many with a label like that. But as long as they're so called and they get away with it, being called antidepressants, they will sell and it doesn't matter what the data show unfortunately. They will remain popular, because it almost seems like a moral imperative if a patient comes to a doctor and is depressed that you give them something called an antidepressant. Why wouldn't you?

One investigation found that two out of three foster children in Texas are on psychotropic medications. One child was on seventeen different medications. Over three hundred children under the age of seven were on psychotropic medications, many on multiple drugs at once. A 2005 study in the *Journal of Child and Adolescent Psychopharmacology* found that 74% of children seen by a psychiatrist are on a psychotropic drug. Half of these kids are taking two or more psychotropic medications at a time. There are no data with kids to show combining two psychiatric drugs are more effective than one.

# Rights Number Six

Patients have a right to monitor their treatment response with patient-rated outcome measures, such as the Beck Depression Inventory instead of the Hamilton Rating Scale. Most of these studies rely on clinician ratings, and there's a reason for that. But, again, I think it's our responsibility to make sure the patients get a say as to how effective the treatment is and we don't just rely on our impressions. Now, some patients have a long list of things that they want to say: [read from cartoon] "I'm making a list of all the things that piss me off." But we still need to ask them. We need to find out not only how effective these medications are, but what sort of side effects they are experiencing.

Juredeini et al (2004) did a wonderful critical review of the published literature on antidepressants in children. Some of these data overlap with what Dr. Healy presented, but it's important and cannot be repeated too much. They found inflated benefits and minimized harm in most of these studies. Half the clinician measures favored the studied drug, but none of the patient or parent measures favored the studied drug in this meta-analysis of randomized controlled trials of antidepressants in kids. The effects were small and of questionable clinical significance. Reliance on questionable statistical practices, which I won't bore you with now, are some of the statistical tricks that Dr. Healy was talking about and are part of the strategy. And, of course, patients are likely to be un-blinded by the side effects (i.e., realize they are not given a placebo by feeling the side effects). In other words, these studies purportedly are double-blind, but that's extremely unlikely. Roger Greenberg did a study some years ago, looking at studies that tested the blind, and in the vast majority of cases, the blind was penetrated by side effects. Patients can tell whether they are on the active drug by the side effects they experience. Clinicians who were doing the ratings can tell. But it's more than that. We educate the patients before the study starts what side effects they could experience on the drug. So we're teaching them how to unblind the study, and that's built into the studies. It's considered standard practice in RCTs. The Keller et al. (2001) study that Dr. Healy mentioned and says should be one of the most famous studies on the planet, randomly assigned 275 children with major depression to Paxil and imipramine, or placebo. Seven children on the Paxil condition had to be hospitalized compared with zero on the placebo condition. But yet they concluded the drug was generally well tolerated in this adolescent population and most adverse events were not serious. So this is an example of what Juredeini points out is minimizing harm. None of the eight outcome measures identified in the original protocol were significantly different among the conditions. The patients in the Paxil condition were six times more likely to develop using what Healy has referred to as euphemistic labeling, "emotional lability," the significance of which was not reported. Some suicidal patients were coded as noncompliant and not included in the data analysis. No wonder Catherine De Angelis et al. (2004), upon noting the prevalence of this kind of stuff, made the following statement: "It is simply no longer possible to believe much of the clinical research that is published or to rely on the judgment of trusted physicians or authoritative medical guidelines. I take no pleasure in this conclusion that I reached slowly and reluctantly over my two decades as editor of the *New England Journal of Medicine*." She is an incredible source, I would say.

The internal document that Healy referred to in his presentation, here it is again, quoting the two passages that make this kind of an internet sensation: "It would be commercially unacceptable to include a statement that efficacy had not been demonstrated as this would undermine the profile of paroxetine..." (in other words, it had not demonstrated the efficacy of Paxil in kids so—and it would hurt the bottom line profit margin, so they could not say that ) "...and no regulatory submissions will be made to obtain either efficacy or safety statements relating to adolescent depression."

How many of you are parents? I'm just curious. Raise your hands. How many of you would be pissed off to know that a drug company was suppressing data about the safety and efficacy of a medicine your kid might take because they were afraid that it might hurt their profit margin? And this is the kind of thing that should make you angry. I'm a parent, too, as I have a 12-year-old. My son, especially when he was little, was an involuntary patient. If he was prescribed something and I was convinced that it was going to help him, I made him take it. And so that's the extra burden we face when we're treating kids.

Patients have a right to untainted scientific data conveyed in a consumer-friendly way regarding psychotropic drugs. I have shown you data, Dr. Healy has shown you data about the distortion in the literature and it comes out in the ads too. In reading them, people might well say: [read from cartoon] "I think the dosage needs adjusting as I'm not nearly as happy as the people in the ads." A former graduate (Amanda Drews) and I, along with Irving Kirsch, (Drews. Antonuccio and Kirsch, in press), looked at the published literature on SSRIs in kids. In the published literature, we found that the placebo duplicated 75% of the effect of the drug. That's quite high. You know, it still looked as if there was some advantage to the drug, at least in the published literature. But in the unpublished studies it shrunk quite a bit, and what clearly is happening here is a publication bias. Studies that show negative effects are less likely to get published. And so our literature is skewed.

I'm going to present again the data of our colleague Erick Turner (2008), because I think this is important. He got the original FDA data because he worked for the FDA, and about half of the studies, the randomized controlled trials for antidepressants showed them to be better than the placebo, but half did not. But as was noted, when you look at the published literature, the weight of the evidence seems to favor antidepressants because, if you relied on the published literature alone, 94% of the antidepressant studies are positive. If you relied on the FDA analysis, that included all the data in theory, it shows that only 51% of the antidepressant studies were positive. Okay? Look at this again. 51% were positive that way. 94% were positive based on the journals.

The journals effectively increased the perceived effect size of the average antidepressant by 32%. Another nuance to these data: 3449 human subjects never had their data published. Of course, what do we tell patients who enroll in our scientific studies? We tell them they're contributing to science. This is in fact probably the most important thing they're doing. Sure. They might earn a few bucks for it, but their data are going to be used to help mankind, humankind, but this analysis that Turner did that was published in the *New England Journal of Medicine* showed that 3449 of these patients volunteered, thinking they were contributing to science, never had their data published. But worse, 1843 human subjects had their data spun in a positive way in contradiction to what the FDA analysis showed. So not only were there many patients whose data were not used, but those who were in trials that showed negative outcomes often had their data published in contrast to the actual findings. Okay? So this is why I think we need this Bill of Rights, and the last item on the Bill of Rights having to do with access to untainted data. Healy and I have written some things in The *British Medical Journal*, advocating that no Internal Review Board approve a study involving human subjects unless there is a commitment to make their data accessible. That is part of the admission price for getting to do a study with human subjects. That's part of your obligation, your moral and ethical obligation that should also be a legal obligation.

Despite all the evidence against the efficacy of antidepressants, they are still as popular as ever: [read from cartoon] "Put him on antidepressants...he just read the reports on their effectiveness." And this is the problem. Despite the overwhelming data about the marginal effectiveness and the significantly increased risk of harm, these medications are going to continue to be prescribed at high levels because they're antidepressants. Why wouldn't you give one if someone is depressed? That's it. Thank you.

# References

Brown, S.A., & Schuckitt, M. (1988). Changes in depression among abstinent alcoholics. *Journal for the Study of Alcoholism, 49,* 412-417.

De Angelis, C., Drazen, J.M., Frizelle, C., et al. (2004). Statement from the International Committee of Medical Journal Editors. *New England Journal of Medicine, 351*(12), 1250-1251.

DeRubeis, R.J., Hollon, S.D., Amsterdam, J.D., Shelton, R.C., Young, P.R., Solomon, R.M., et al. (2005). Cognitive therapy vs. medications in the treatment of moderate to severe depression. *Archives of General Psychiatry, 62,* 409-416.

Drews, A., Antonuccio, D.O, & Kirsch, I. (2011). A meta-analysis of randomized placebo controlled trials of antidepressant medications in depressed children weighing the benefits and risks. *Journal of Mind-Body Regulation, 1*(2), 31-41.

Greenberg, R.P. (2002). Reflections on the Emperors New Drugs. *Prevention and Treatment, 27,* 17-19.

Hollon, S.D., DeRubeis, R.C., Shelton, R.C., & Weiss, B. (2005). The Emperor's New Drugs: Effect size and moderation effects. *Prevention and Treatment, 5, Article 27.*

Jureidini, J.N., Doecke, C.J., Mansfield, P.R., Haby, M.M., Menkes, D.B., & Tonkin, A.L. (2004). Efficacy and safety of antidepressants for Children and adolescents. *British Medical Journal, 328,* 79-883.

Keller, M., Montgomery, S., Ball, W. et al (2001). Efficacy of Paroxetine in the treatment of adolescent major depression: A randomized, controlled trial. *Journal of the American Academy of Child and Adolescent Psychiatry, 40*(7), 762-772.

Kirsch, I. (2010). *The emperor's new drugs.* New York: Basic Books.

Koran, L.M., Bullock, K.D., Hartston, H.J., Elliott, M.A., & D'Andrea, V. (2002). Medical disorders among patients admitted to a public-sector psychiatric inpatient unit. *Psychiatric Services,* December, *53*(12), 1623-1625.

Treatment for Adolescents with Depression Study (TADS) Team, (2004). Fluoxetine, cognitive –behavioral therapy, and their combination for adolescents with depression. *Journal of the American Medical Association, 292,* 807-820.

Treatment for Adolescents with Depression Study (TADS) Team, (2007). Long-term effectiveness and safety outcomes. *Archives of General Psychiatry, 64,* 1132-1144.

Turner, E.H., Matthews, A.M., Linardatos, E., et al. (2008). Selective publication of antidepressant trials and its influence on apparent efficacy. *New England Journal of Medicine, 358,* 252-260.

Chapter 4

# Psychotherapy as the First Line Treatment for Behavioral Disorders:

*Treatments, Outcomes, and Cost Effectiveness*

*John Caccavale, Ph.D., ABMP*
*National Alliance of Professional Psychology Providers*

## Introduction

My presentation today focuses on the comparative effectiveness of psychotherapy and behavioral interventions on behavioral disorders. Clearly, a topic well-suited to this conference. However, comparative effectiveness is not a uni-dimensional assessment. A simple "did Group A do better than Group B" can provide only a sliver of whether a treatment is effective. Healthcare providers are constantly faced with study after study touting the benefits of some new drug, a new procedure, a new therapy or new look at something previously used. With respect to drugs, numbers are always misleading. For example, a study may show that drug A is about 40% more effective than drug B. On the surface, it would appear that drug B is less effective. However, upon further analysis, the reported effectiveness in the reduction of symptoms shows the "effectiveness" to be only 3% to 2% better. Although the treatment effect is small and really insignificant, the manufacturer can claim a whopping increase in effectiveness. This is a common and frequent occurrence in medicine.

Medications account for hundreds of billions of dollars in the overall healthcare budget. Outcomes without a relationship to reduced costs obscures the real and significant impact that psychotherapy as a first line treatment has on healthcare policy. An analysis of what treatments work best and their costs can shed new light on why the medicalization of behavioral health has proven to be more a function of the power of drug manufacturers than to the available science on medications and an economic analysis of their worth and effectiveness. The goal of this presentation is to examine the relationships between a representative group of the most frequently occurring behavioral disorders, the most effective demonstrated treatments for them and the costs associated with providing these treatments. An analysis of the important data shows that having an appropriate diagnosis and treatment from a trained behavioral health provider is more effective and cost efficient when compared to treatment with psychotropic medications. Moreover, if behavioral strategies were to be used more frequently and concurrently with the five most frequent medical conditions (diabetes mellitus, heart disease, metabolic syndrome, cancer and respiratory problems), overall patient health would increase as total healthcare costs decrease.

## Costs For Medication Treatments

Between the years 1996 and 2006, expenditures for behavioral health treatment rose from $35.2 billion in 1996 to 57.5 billion in 2006. By 2009, the total expenditure for mental healthcare amounted to about 4% of total healthcare expenditures of $2.2 trillion dollars, or about $100 billion dollars.[1] This increase in expenditures is directly related to the expanded use of psychotropic medications and to the shift of behavioral healthcare to primary care physicians. The shift to primary care has led to misdiagnoses and non-treatment of behavioral health disorders. The result of this shift clearly can be associated with poor health outcomes and increased healthcare costs. On the other side of this issue, but one that is less likely to be reported, is the impact of an appropriate diagnosis and treatment of behavioral health disorders on reducing total healthcare expenditures.

For calendar year 2009, total sales of prescription medications exceeded $300 billion dollars.[2] And this does not include over-the-counter sales of wildly claimed herbals and vitamins. The net effect and clinical significance of medications is that, increasingly, fewer people are benefited from many medication interventions. For example, statin medications are the second most common class of drugs that are prescribed.[2] Yet, study after study shows that the big gainers from these drugs are people who already have experienced a heart attack. People who are healthy with no known cardiac symptoms or significant risks, but have high cholesterol, are not helped by statins. Yet, physicians and medical guidelines continue to press people to use them. Statins account for billions of dollars in sales. Billions down the drain and many people are left with side effects from these drugs as their only "benefit". Moreover, behavioral interventions to help patients adhere to better diets, exercise and other lifestyle programs, are so infrequently prescribed, yet can be much more effective than these drugs and far less costly over the life of the patient.

Psychotropic medications, on the other hand, year after year, continue to see big gains in overall prescriptions written and increases in sales. For example, for the 2009 calendar year, the number of prescriptions written for antipsychotic medications exceeded 52 million producing sales of $14.6 billion dollars. In fact, sales of antipsychotics were the number one medication in overall sales for 2009 replacing statin medications.[2] Clearly, antipsychotic medication are being over prescribed off label for non-psychotic conditions despite the potential dangerous side effects for these drugs. The retail costs for the four most frequently prescribed psychotropic medications for the year 2009 account for 40% of the total expenditure for mental health services excluding other treatment services related to substance abuse. It is expected that retail sales for 2010 will see about a 10% increase over 2009. The point here is that 40% of the national mental healthcare budget goes to drug treatments that, for the most part, have not been proven to be any more effective than placebo and certainly not more effective than psychotherapeutic interventions.

In a comparative study of the costs of selective psychotropic medications (source: *IMS International Sales Perspective)* for calendar year 2009 reveals total sales as follows: Antipsychotics, 14,6 billion. Antidepressants (SSRIs and SNRIs only, excluding tricyclics and MAOI classes of antidepressants, 9.9 billion. Anxiolytics, 8.9 billion Anticonvulsants, 5.3 billion. The total for just these "mental health" drugs is 34.7 billion, or approximately one-tenth of the total U.S. pharmaceutical budget.

A recent study shows that there is measurable brain shrinkage as a result of taking these medications.[3] Antipsychotics are being prescribed for sleep disorders, depression, and anxiety. All of which respond positively to psychotherapy and behavioral intervention. So the question becomes: Is it worth experiencing Extra Pyramidal Symptoms, such as pseudoparkinsonism, tardive dyskinesia, and brain shrinkage when psychotherapy is so much more effective for these non-psychotic conditions and with little to none side effects? I think not.

# Determining Which Person Will Benefit From Which Intervention

Given the costs of useless medications and procedures, it would seem that a better approach would be to identify which patients would benefit from a specific treatment. This approach requires rational decisions when selecting treatment options, but does raise significant social, ethical, and political issues. Should a person who doesn't fit the profile be denied a medication? How effective are the profiles used to identify potential beneficiaries? Would it be a denial of constitutional rights to deny a drug or service? These are questions that can rightly be raised. However, these questions may also be irrelevant to the issue. This means subscribing to providing the right treatment, by the right person, and at the right time.

The issue is not to deny a drug or service, but to stop using a shotgun approach and using a scientifically valid approach to treatment. Why provide a statin to a person who has no risk factors aside from high cholesterol? Should not these people be provided behavioral intervention and lifestyle changes such as exercising and reducing their intake of sugar, saturated fats, and empty calories, which is more related to higher levels of cholesterol? Why should narcotic pain medications be provided to patients when so many can learn how to reduce their pain by other means such as biofeedback and relaxation exercises? Why should antipsychotic medications be prescribed to people who have a sleep disturbance when behavioral interventions are the first line treatment for this problem? There are so many other examples that there is little room to accommodate them in such a short presentation.

# The Effectiveness Of Psychotherapy As A First Line Treatment

Although some of us would like to believe that all psychological interventions are effective—they are not. And, when treatment doesn't work, it may not be because the treatment is invalid, but simply inappropriate for that patient and a specific diagnosis. For example, some practitioners still rely on many therapies that are not based on any real scientific research. There is a whole school of therapy that is based on the notion that "the apple doesn't fall far from the tree." Another, has as its main tenet: "I think therefore I am." While these approaches may be fine for some patients, there is no dispute that the many adherents of these therapies tend to treat all their patients with the same perspective. The result is wasted opportunities for real change and a really high cost to benefit ratio. So, psychologists, too, will need to address these issues post healthcare reform.

Several years ago, J. Allan Hobson wrote a book called *Out of its Mind: Psychiatry in Crisis*.[4] Although a critique of psychiatry, psychology is also called to task. Hobson makes the point that as psychiatry abandoned therapy, it became mindless. This left people to be treated by drugs or treated by medically ignorant psychologists, who Hobson called "brainless," because of our insufficient knowledge of brain functioning. Today, although many psychologists are much more sophisticated about biological processes and possess extensive psychopharmacological training and expertise, most of us still remain, in Hobson's term, "brainless". Post healthcare reform will only bring greater focus to this problem.

# Psychotherapy For Treating Depression Is Effective And Cost Efficient

Depression is a major behavioral disorder and one that is both costly and ineffectively treated when using medications as a first line treatment.[5-7] It is no secret that the pharmaceutical industry is garnering huge profits and is likely to make even more under healthcare reform. Among the most profitable and growing segment of pharmaceuticals are psychotropic medications. For example, in 1996, the industry, as a whole, spent $32 million on direct-to-consumer (DTC) antidepressant advertising.[6] By 2005, that number grew to $122 million. See, advertising does work! In excess of 164 million antidepressant prescriptions were written in 2009, totaling $10 billion in U.S. sales.[2] Today, whether in the ubiquitous television ads or in magazines, consumers are being extolled to tell their physicians the name and type of medication that they want. Physicians, for the most part, willingly respond. Yet, with respect to antidepressants, the latest science casts great doubt that there is any significant difference between any of the SSRI medications and, moreover, whether they really work as advertised.[6,7] One obvious question is whether the ads are driving the incidence rate of depression or is greater awareness of depression driving the increasing number of prescriptions? The answer to this question is important not only for its clinical significance, but also because it is important to the economics of healthcare reform.

One could make the case that depression is being diagnosed more frequently today than a decade ago because of greater public awareness and because primary care physicians have become the first line providers of mental healthcare. However, study after study shows that primary care physicians, as a group, lack the expertise to diagnose depression as well as other mental disorders.[8] In fact, patients who are clinically depressed receive about 50% of the standard of care that organized medicine requires in their treatment guidelines.[9] And, not just by mere coincidence, patients who are clinically depressed typically go for several years before getting the appropriate diagnosis and treatment from primary care physicians. Now, this does not mean that primary care physicians are bad people or incompetent. Most are not. The problem is that they just aren't skilled mental health specialists and, problematically, the "training" they do get, typically comes in the form of a young drug sales representative.

On the other hand, why would an industry quadruple its advertising budget for a single class of drug if advertising was ineffective? These are not new facts, but they are relevant. Psychotropic medications are proliferating. I call this the "Cerealization of Medications." The marketing strategy is no different than that employed by cereal manufacturers who line supermarket shelves with tens of boxes of the same sugar-laden cereals. It's called getting and holding market share. Patients are being prescribed unnecessary medications and not getting the appropriate treatment because behavioral health specialists are being kept out of the treatment mix and because pills, in the short term only, are cheaper than behavioral care.

Major Depressive Disorder is a serious and debilitating condition. The prevalence rate reported by the Agency for Healthcare Research and Quality (AHRQ) for adults age 18 and over with serious psychological distress in the past year was 24.3 million.[10] Adults age 18 and over with a major depressive episode during the year 2007 was 16.5 million.[10] Adults with at least one major depressive episode in their lifetime was 30.4 million.[11] The AHRQ estimates that the direct and indirect costs to treatment depression, based on 2003 figures, was about $130 billion dollars. The direct treatment cost was about $25 billion dollars. Antidepressant medications accounted for $10 billion dollars for 2009. Another $5 billion dollars accounted for hospitalizations. This leaves about $10 billion dollars that can be ascribed to behavioral treatment for depression.

Treatment with medications only is now considered a lifelong therapy. Treatment with psychotherapy and behavioral intervention, in most cases, is time limited. So while initial costs for psychotherapy may be greater, long term costs are finite. Moreover, medication only treatments require other medically related services such as frequent blood panels and office visits. Over the life of the patient, cost efficiency can hardly be a selling point for medication regimens. The least attractive part of medication only regimens is that there are no cures. Among those patients who report that medications have improved their condition, once off medications brings a return to their depression. This is why these medications are a lifelong treatment. Patients learn no new coping skills from medications. There is no neurogenesis as that which occurs with learning new coping skills. So, even if one can match dollar for dollar, psychotherapy is far more effective and cost efficient than a medication only approach to treatment.

The best available research tells us that psychotherapy is an effective and cost efficient treatment for depression. For example, as early as 1990, a review of the literature confirms that depressed patients benefit substantially from psychotherapy, and these gains appear comparable or better than those observed with pharmacotherapy.[12] A 2007 study showed that psychotherapy for depression was an effective treatment for 80% of the patients studied. When used in combination with medications, several studies conclude that the combination is more effective than medications alone.[13] For patients who have shown resistance to treatment with medications, psychotherapy appears to be an equally effective treatment compared to antidepressant medication and is therefore a reasonable treatment option.[14] The case for psychotherapy, I believe, is clear cut.

## Anxiety Disorders

Anxiety disorders are the most prevalent psychiatric conditions in the United States, aside from disorders involving substance abuse. Generalized anxiety disorder has a lifetime prevalence of 5%. Anxiety disorders include panic disorder, obsessive-compulsive disorder, post-traumatic stress disorder, generalized anxiety disorder, and phobias (social phobia, agoraphobia, and specific phobia). Approximately 40 million American adults ages 18 and older, or about 18.1% of people in this age group in a given year, have an anxiety disorder. Anxiety disorders frequently co-occur with depressive disorders or substance abuse. Most people with one anxiety disorder also have another anxiety disorder. Nearly three-quarters of those with an anxiety disorder will have their first episode by age 21.[15]

In an early article reviewing the various treatments for Panic Disorder with Agoraphobia (PDA), the researchers concluded that cognitive-behavioral therapy was a most effective treatment for PDA. Their conclusion was based on comparisons of CBT and medication treatments. The review of approximately 150 research studies showed that 87% of people with PDA improved with only a 10% relapse rate for CBT as compared to a 60% improvement rate with a 35% relapse rate for anti-depressants and a 60% improvement rate with a 90% relapse rate for anti-anxiety medications. CBT for Panic Disorder without Agoraphobia has an improvement rate of 90% with a 5% relapse rate.[16]

In a 2010, study published in the *Journal of the American Medical Association*, the authors compared the effectiveness of a combination of CBT along with other evidenced-based treatments against medications. The participants consisted of 1004 patients with varying anxiety disorders including panic, generalized anxiety, social anxiety, and post-traumatic stress disorder in 17 primary care clinics in 4 U.S. cities. Patients were seen in follow-up visits after 6, 12, and 18 months. Results showed that behavioral interventions were significantly more effective than any other types of treatment, including medications, in reducing global anxiety symptoms. These patients also experienced higher response and remission rates. [17, 22]

Contrasting behavioral interventions with medications for anxiety disorders results in a clear cut choice. The typical medication regimen of treating with benzodiazepines produces sedation and is highly addictive. The treatment regimen is also life-long. I might add that in my practice, where I have treated many patients for a wide range of anxiety disorders, the most treatment resistant patients were those on long term benzodiazepines such as Lorazapam. High costs for treatments typically is not the in the cost of medications, but in the high volume of office visits and general high maintenance of patients presenting with anxiety disorders. Behavioral intervention with CBT, for example, typically consists of 13–16 sessions and cost generally in the range of $1300 to $2400 dollars. Many other approaches, such as Exposure Therapy, Dialectic Behavior Therapy and Interpersonal Therapy, have also been effective and cost efficient treatments. On the other side, for fiscal year 2007, the costs to treat anxiety disorders with medications was $9 billion dollars.[2] Once again, the myth and misplaced notion that medications are a real first line treatment for behavioral disorders simply is not supported by the data. In terms of treatment effectiveness and cost efficiency, psychotherapy and other behavioral interventions are the real first line treatments.[23]

## The Five Most Costly Medical Conditions

I would now like to address the relationship between behavioral interventions and medical disorders. In terms of healthcare expenditures, five medical conditions are ranked as the most costly conditions between 1996 and 2006, when most official estimates are reported. When comparing these illnesses over time, there was an increase in the expenditures for each of these conditions. The "Big Five" most costly conditions were: cardiac disease, respiratory disorders, cancer, metabolic disorders, and mental disorders. During this period, the largest increase in expenditures was for mental disorders and trauma-related disorders. The expenditures for mental disorders, excluding nursing care and hospitalizations, rose from $35.2 billion in 1996 (in 2006 dollars) to 57.5 billion in 2006.[18]

With respect to cardiac disease, in 2009, the treatment of cardiac related-disorders and disease, according to the American Heart Association, was $183 billion dollars.[19] The total projected cost for cancer related treatment is about $84 billion dollars for fiscal year 2010.[19] Presently, about 4% of healthcare dollars are spent on the overall direct costs related to diabetes. This amounts to about to $92 billion a year. The Centers for Disease Control and Prevention predicts that spending on diabetes care will reach $192 billion in 2020.[20] The cost of treating chronic respiratory disease is predicted to more than double from $176.8 billion in 2006 to $389.2 billion in 2011.

The alarming part of all this should not be focused on the high amount of expenditures for these diseases, but on the fact that much of these conditions can be effectively treated with behavioral interventions at sizable savings and with relatively few, if any, side effects. Moreover, for many people who are diagnosed with these conditions behavioral intervention may be the best way to improve their overall health. For example, a large part of cardiac disorders are related to lifestyle decisions. Poor diet, little exercise, and poor attitude and decision making contribute to overweight and obesity. Much of the same can be said about diabetes. Many people suffering from respiratory disorders are greatly improved through respiratory rehab programs that teach proper breathing techniques, diet, exercise, and stress reduction. Further, the conditions of many of these patients experience co-morbid mental disorders including depression and anxiety, to name a few. With the combination of appropriate lifestyle medical care and behavioral intervention these patients experience better health while reducing overall healthcare costs.[21]

Thus, it is not farfetched to conclude that a significant reduction in overall healthcare costs can be achieved if treatments included behavioral interventions and psychotherapy. Even a small 10% reduction would equal the whole mental health budget to say nothing of the improvement in both the physical and mental health of the patients who suffer from these disorders. The use of behavioral health specialists, those trained in applying behavioral interventions to medical problems, can be and are an effective solution to control the unnecessary rise and subsequent costs for psychotropic and other classes of medications. Speaking out against the proliferation and overuse of medications is wise advocacy. Our training as behavioral health specialists allows us to diagnose mental disorders quickly and accurately and we provide effective and efficient behavioral interventions when included in the treatment process. Treatments that rely on medications result in increased use and increased costs for medications, but at a cost for less effective treatment for patients.

So why have we been left out of the mix? Primarily, we are left out because we do not have control over the treatment process, which I will discuss further when we have our friendly debate. Secondly, the bulk of healthcare dollars go to physicians. Thirdly, organized medicine resists real collaboration with other professionals who seek expansion in their scope of practice, perceived or real. Fourth, the economics of medications is a $300 billion industry. Drug manufacturers can manipulate data, buy research results, and buy political power. Lastly, mental health providers are a fragmented group of professions that also resists organizing even if that would result in greater power to get the message to patients and to policymakers. Over the past 30 years our organizational efforts have been devoted to minimizing cuts to the mental health budget. An activity, I might add, that has been a failure. Finally, our colleague, Dr. Nicholas Cummings, has repeatedly demonstrated that psychotherapy is an effective and cost efficient treatment for behavioral problems.[24, 25] We need to keep repeating this message as it needs to be heard again and again.

# References

1.  Stagnitti, M. N. ( 2009). *Trends in the Use and Expenditures for the Therapeutic Class Prescribed Psychotherapeutic Agents and All Subclasses, 1996 and 2008.* Statistical Brief #163. February 2009. Rockville, MD: Agency for Healthcare Research and Quality.

2.  IMS HEALTH, Top Therapeutic Classes by U.S. Sales. April 2010. http://imshealth.com.

3.  Beng-Choon, H, Andreasen, NC, Ziebell, S, Pierson, R, Magnotta, V. (2011). **A Longitudinal Study of First-Episode Schizophrenia. Arch Gen Psychiatry.** 2011; 68(2):128-137. doi:10.1001/archgenpsychiatry.2010.199.

4.  Hobson, JA, Leonard, JA. (2002). Out Of Its Mind: Psychiatry in Crisis: A Call for Reform. Cambridge, Mass., Perseus Publishing.

5.  Kirsch, I., Moore, T., Scoboria, A., & Nichols, S. (2002). The emperor's new drugs: An analysis of antidepressant medication data submitted to the U.S. Food and Drug Administration. *Prevention and Treatment, 5,* 23. Retrieved March 2004, http://journals.apa.org/prevention/volume5/pre0050025e.html

6.  Caccavale, JL. Caccavale, J. (2010). Failure to serve: the misuse of medications as first line treatments for behavioral disorders. http://nappp.org/White_paper.pdf

7.  Antonuccio, D.O., Burns, D., & Danton, W.G. (2002). Antidepressants: A triumph of marketing over science? *Prevention and Treatment, 5,* Article 25. Available on the World Wide Web: http://www.journals.apa.org/prevention/volume5/pre0050025c.html.

8.  Klinkman, M.S. & Okkes, I. (1998). Mental health problems in primary care: a research agenda. *Journal of Family Practice, 47,* 379-384.

9.  McGlyn, EA., Asch, SM., Adams, J., Keesey, J., Hicks, J., Cristofaro, A., & Kerr, EA. (2003).The quality of healthcare delivered to adults in the United States. *The New England Journal of Medicine,* 348, 26, 2635-2645

10. Substance Abuse and Mental Health Services Administration. Results from the 2007 National Survey on Drug Use and Health: national findings. Rockville, MD: Office of Applied Studies; 2008. NSDUH Series H-34. Publication No. SMA 08-4343.

11. Substance Abuse and Mental Health Services Administration. Results from the 2006 National Survey on Drug Use and Health: national findings. Rockville, MD: Office of Applied Studies; 2007. NSDUH Series H-32. Publication No. 07-4293. Rockville, MD: Office of Applied Studies; 2006.

12. Robinsona, LA, Berman, JS, & Neimeyer, RA. (1990). Psychotherapy for the Treatment of Depression: A Comprehensive Review of Controlled Outcome Research *Psychological Bulletin*, Volume 108, Issue 1, July 1990, Pages 30-49.

13. Arnow BA, Constantino MJ. (2003). Aug; 59(8):893-905.Effectiveness of psychotherapy and combination treatment for chronic depression. *J Clin Psychol*, Aug; 59(8):893-905.

14. Department of Veterans Affairs. Evidence Synthesis for Determining the Efficacy of Psychotherapy for Treatment Resistant Depression. Oct 2009.

15. Kessler RC, Chiu WT, Demler O, Walters EE. Prevalence, severity, and comorbidity of twelve-month DSM-IV disorders in the National Comorbidity Survey Replication (NCS-R). *Archives of General Psychiatry*, 2005 Jun; 62(6):617-27.

16. Michelson, L.K. & Marchione, K. (1991). Behavioral, Cognitive, and Pharmacological Treatments of PDA: Critique and Synthesis. *Journal of Consulting and Clinical Psychology*, 59, 100-114.

17. Roy-Byrne, P., Craske, M. G., Sullivan, G., Rose, R. D., Edlund, M. J., Lang, A. J., Bystritsky, A., Welch, S. S., Chavira, D. A., Golinelli, D., Campbell-Sills, L., Sherbourne, C. D., & Stein, M. B. (2010). Delivery of evidence-based treatment for multiple anxiety disorders in primary care. *The Journal of the American Medical Association*, 303, 1921-1928.

18. Soni, A. (2009). *The Five Most Costly Conditions, 1996 and 2006: Estimates for the U.S. Civilian Noninstitutionalized Population*. Statistical Brief #248. July 2009. Agency for Healthcare Research and Quality, Rockville, MD.

19. The Hasting Center. Cost Trends in Heart Disease, End Stage Renal Disease, Cancer, and Metabolic Syndrome. May 22, 2009.

20. Hastings Center. The Projected cost of Chronic Disease. January, 2010.

21. Golubic, M. (2011). Comparative Efficacy of Lifestyle Practices for Certain Chronic Conditions, Comparison of Medications with Lifestyle Medicine. ACPM conference Feb 17, 2011.
22. Anxiety and Mood Disorders: Use and Expenditures for Adults 18 and Older, U.S. Civilian Noninstitutionalized Population, 2007 Medical Expenditure Panel Survey. December 2010.
23. *Evid Based Mental Health.* (2010). **13:79 doi:10.1136/ ebmh.13.3.79** A GP training package for the treatment of anxiety disorders is not cost-effective.
24. Cummings, NA, O'Donohue, WT, & Cummings, JL. (2009). The Financial Dimension of Integrated Behavioral/Primary Care. *Journal of Clinical Psychology in Medical Settings*, DOI 10.1007/ s10880-008-9139-2
25. Cummimgs, N.A., Dorken, H., Pallak, M. S., & Henke, C. (1990). *The impact of psychological intervention on healthcare untilizationand costs.* South San Francisco: The Biodyne Institute.

Chapter 5

# Moderated Discussion: Psychotherapy as a First Line Treatment

*A Panel Discussion with John Caccavale, Ph.D. and David Anto-nuccio, Ph.D.,*

*with William O'Donohue, Ph.D. as Moderator*

DR. O'DONOHUE (MODERATOR): First, I thought we'd allow the two panelists to react to each other's talk. So David and John, are there any comments you want to make about each other's talk, any things that you disagree with? We'd like, you know, to get some lively debate. If you're in entire agreement, would you like to talk about each other's mothers?

DOCTOR CACCAVALE: David and I have had conversations in the past about these issues, and I like approaches that are more than two dimensions or one dimensional. And I agree 100% with David's Patient Bill of Rights. But, you know, he started off by talking about the Bill of Rights that we have in our Constitution, but people are still fighting for those rights. And so "rights" to me don't necessarily translate into getting the kinds of actions that we want, and even though that's not what he's saying. It's not a criticism that he's saying stop at the Bill of Rights, but what I'm saying is that we need to take those Bill of Rights and translate them into activities that become standards that providers need to abide by.

For example, while David looks at his Bill of Rights, I have developed a corollary set of standards. In fact, Dr. Cummings, myself, and another colleague have just written a paper on that. There is one thing that we'd like to see enforced with respect to psychotropic drugs, and although it also applies to other classes also, I'm at this point just talking about psychotropic drugs. There should be no off-label prescribing. If the research is not supporting drugs that have been approved, then you can't certainly subject a patient to unapproved drugs. That makes no sense whatsoever. And there should be no polypharmacy beyond two medications, because we haven't seen anything that supports that. And the reason why it is important to be looking at the polypharmacy issue and the off-label issue , is that drug companies are now marketing two drugs in one pill.

So we need to do that, but we also need to be able to say that, as a standard, a patient who goes into primary care and there's no mental health practitioner co-located, which is the preference that we have, then the patient has to be provided with a set of options. That's the standard, not only as their right, but that needs to be the provider's standard as well. There's a whole number of these standards that we've outlined that really go along with David's Bill of Rights. How come we're so close on that? Is that because we're both Italian! No, that's not the reason, even though that may partly be the reason, I suspect.

We actually were trying to put together these standards and the Patient Bill of Rights together in one place. But we found it kind of difficult. And so we decided that, being good colleagues, he'll write about patient rights and I'll write about standards. I wouldn't say this constitutes a disagreement. What I'm saying is that I just think that unless providers are forced to provide appropriately, patients can have all the rights in the world, but even under the U.S. Constitution, I have people saying: I may have rights, but I have to go to court in order to get them. So "rights" to me are just too watered down.

The other thing that I have a problem with is that when a patient is feeling ill, they are looking towards this person called the physician, or called the therapist, or whatever, and they're not thinking about rights. This is because if they were able to think about rights, they would see they do not belong there. If they knew about all the rights, they probably wouldn't be there in the first place. Rather, they would be seeing the appropriate person. So, again, it's not a disagreement. It's just that I just think that we have to take what David is talking about and we have to make those into standards that we can enforce upon providers.

DOCTOR ANTONUCCIO: You know, Caccavale and Antonuccio, if this meeting were taking place in Nevada, the Nevada Gaming Control Board would want to get an intervener or something.

I have been training psychiatrists for 30 years, and that's why I have kind of lost faith in our ability to shape the prescribers' behavior. I've worked with some wonderful psychiatry residents and continue to do so, along with wonderful psychiatric colleagues. Yet I don't feel like the impact on prescribing practices has been very great, honestly, and so that's part of the problem.

The other issue for me is in terms of prescription privileges for psychologists. I will say that I agree with 90% probably of the stuff that you present, and the data you present, so there's a very small well of disagreements. So I don't know how much of a debate this will be per se. But in terms of prescribing privileges, my feeling has been clear, but I've never publicly opposed prescribing privileges because it would feel too disloyal to the psychologists who choose to pursue that.

But from my perspective, the tools we seek are not as good as the tools we already have, and so I feel like putting our energy in that area is not where I want to put my efforts. So my feeling is, with this Patient Bill of Rights, it is just one way to empower patients to demand the kind of treatments I think they deserve and that are supported by the data. I just don't feel like we are having much impact on the providers. I've been at this for a long time, since 1995 really. I've been writing about this sort of thing with minimal impact, I think, except for a small group of folks.

DOCTOR CACCAVALE: I've been a proponent of prescriptive authority for psychologists from the very beginning, going back to 1990, 1989, 1988, something like that. I'm also formally trained as a psychopharmacologist. I have a postdoctoral degree in psychopharmacology. And why do I support that? Seemingly, it is a paradox to what you've heard me say. And, in fact, the things that I write about would also seem to be a paradox. But they really aren't. And here's why.

Who would you rather be treated by or your patient or your family be treated by? It is a primary care physician, because that's really what the option is right now. You will go to see that person who will spend very few minutes with you, who in all probability will give you an erroneous diagnosis if at all, will provide you with a treatment that is ineffective and perhaps even harmful, and will be quite unresponsive in terms of the needs that you have as patient. If you have a depression or other behavioral health issue, would you not rather be treated by a psychologist who has prescriptive authority, and who looks at medications in the same way that you heard us talk about it today? For example, to be treated by someone who knows that very few people under very strict conditions are helped by medications? Or, give you the option of behavior treatment first by a person who is quite aware of the research surrounding not only the behavioral treatment, but also the medications? Which person would you prefer seeing on a regular basis?

To me, that's a no-brainer, because I've trained psychiatrists also for six years at UCLA. We have had the same experiences, and I can say that I came across one psychiatrist with whom I became a very close personal friend that was actually the anti-psychiatrist to become friends with. The fact remains, we have a system as it is right now that needs to be changed. We are in a very difficult position in terms of making those changes. But if we're looking for a solution, it is to have a co-located mental health specialist in primary care. This is what we've been saying for years on end, and I'll continue to campaign for that. But we've not been able to do that. Prescriptive authority turns out to be really one of the solutions that even Dr. Healy talks about. The long history with psychologists who do prescribe shows that not only do psychologists prescribe the least number of medications, but we adhere to the kinds of things that you're talking about here. In fact, even without training, I'm willing to bet you that most psychologists and most of you who practice, the patients that come to you who are on medication, somehow you get them off those medications. That was always one of my goals. And I have accomplished those goals.

In fact, I have been prescribing for years. How have I been doing it? I'm surrounded by physicians who know that they don't do a good job, so they say: Hey, John, let me have your recommendation. Many psychologists have been doing that for years without putting their name on the script. And so it's very important, if we're looking for more effective solutions, to have psychologists apply for prescriptive authority. We're addressing lawmakers, we're addressing policymakers, and we're addressing physicians, and we're saying: This is the reason why we need to prescribe, because it's more cost effective as split treatment models do not work. Integrated care would work if in fact we could get integrated care. That would certainly be a big improvement. But it certainly would not be as much of an improvement if you were even co-located, but someone else is still writing the script. So what we're looking at is this: Which group is really the best group to be dealing with these kinds of issues? And the answer turns out to be that psychologists who are trained in clinical psychopharmacology and medical psychology are really the best equipped.

If we were able to do that, many of the problems that you've heard today would be vastly diminished. Having written three bills already for prescriptive authority, I can tell you that this issue about off-label prescribing should be made part of the statute. Why? There's no reason to give a psychologist or any other provider prescriptive authority under the present system where all they can do is write a script. There's got to be boundaries, and the boundaries should be based on what we know in terms of data-driven versus evidence-driven evidence. And that is, by the way, a very important distinction. The evidence turns out to be not so much the actual evidence. And so it's very, very important that we distinguish ourselves from every other provider. I've been writing about this for years in terms of, what comprises the prescribing psychologist? What is required of the prescribing psychologist are all the things that you've heard here today. You adhere to what we know is the best available science. You do not look at medications as a first-line treatment. You do not engage with off-label prescribing. You do not engage in polypharmacy. You do not engage in foisting upon patients the treatment that you like. You must give the patient options.

So you put these things in the statute that gives the prescriptive authority and now that doesn't mean that someone is not going to violate that. But I can tell you, we've had psychologists prescribing in the military since 1990. We have two states that they're prescribing in right now, and we have hundreds of psychologists who are prescribing under contract to the military. We can go back to Nick's experience in American Biodyne, where in fact the psychologists were handling all the medication issues. And I don't know if you've read his early stuff, but I think it's good reading if you haven't because we keep on citing it.

The matter is that the patients that went to see the psychologists that worked for Nick and also were supervised in Kaiser there, their clinicians' medications was small. As I recall, if they went to the psychiatrist, about 87% of them wound up with a prescription. If they went to the psychologist and went through that route, 67% were off of it. Now, that's what we're talking about as an unbelievable result and an appropriate result.

So, as a psychologist, we already have that experience, and I can tell you, I was never so much against medications in my life until I got trained in them. It's just the opposite with a physician. The more the physician gets training, the more medications they believe in, because they're trained to deal with symptoms. If you've got a symptom, you get medication. Symptom, medication. Symptom, medication.

I'm not saying that this is the best solution. The best solution would be what everybody's been talking about today; that is, to have an ideal system. But that ideal system would mean that you would not be relying upon the kind of for-profit healthcare that makes it profitable to be giving these ineffective drugs. We are referring to the $300 billion cost here, and if we do nothing it will grow to $400 billion and then to $500 billion as we continue to prescribe ineffective treatment treatments that are based on data that shows their effectiveness. But I don't believe that we're going to change that system, so we need to have a solution. And the solution to me is prescriptive authority, because, again, you're not getting appropriate treatment in primary care, and that's where mental health treatment has been transferred.

DOCTOR O'DONOHUE: Your reaction, Dave?

DOCTOR ANTONUCCIO: Yes, two comments and then I think we should open it up to the audience and let them ask some questions.

Two things that give me pause and worry me a little bit. One is that psychiatrists used to do psychotherapy, but the contingencies are such they've been steered in the direction of prescribing pills. So many of you saw the recent article in *The New York Times* probably interviewing this one psychiatrist about his 10-minute meetings with patients and he doesn't have time to ask them about their lives, and if they want to talk about their lives, he has to refer them somewhere else. But that did not used to be the case. And I believe the psychiatry behavior has been shaped by contingencies that are out there, and I think we're subject to the same learning principles as psychologists if we prescribe. That's one issue that concerns me.

The other one is, I participated on a couple of panels at the American Psychological association (APA) convention with prescribing psychologists as part of the Psychopharmacology Division's program. Maybe I shouldn't have been, but I was surprised to find a couple of prescribers using multiple medications even with kids. I think, John, you're probably one of the most careful, prudent prescribers out there. Their justification was that they didn't at first appreciate how severely disturbed some of these kids were and why multiple medications were necessary. So I thought I saw this going along in the same direction that I had seen psychiatry go. The other thing was that one of the prescribers told me that his waiting room looked like a pharmaceutical ad because there were so many emotional things in his waiting room. And so I thought, uh-oh, you know, this is already happening while we're trying to be careful. And so these are the things that worry

DOCTOR CACCAVALE: I'd like to answer that. Again, I've written three bills and I've tried to get even other states that are thinking about prescriptive authority to use these as a model. In

every one of the bills that I wrote, as part of the statute, a prescribing psychologist could not have a practice that was based upon
psychopharmacology. No more than 30% of that practice could
be in psychopharmacology. That really takes care of that issue.
The problem is that we have a model for prescribing now that is
just as we've said: There's no difference right now among anyone
who prescribes because those standards are not there, so they're
not being enforced as part of the statute. You're absolutely right. If
we maintain a system where all you have is a script, at some point
it's going to become a lot easier just to write that script, make a
lot more money seeing a lot more patients on a 10-minute basis. I
share that concern. In order to make sure that that doesn't happen,
you have to codify it in the statute and say that you cannot have a
practice that is purely on the basis of psychopharmacology.

Now, do we have precedents for that? Yes, we do. For example, in California if you're doing disability or workers' compensation evaluations, you cannot have a practice that's full-time
evaluation. Only a small part of that can be for evaluation. You
cannot be 100% into evaluations. Why? Because insurers and
lawyers are often paying for these evaluations, and in essence are
"buying" them. So you must see patients and you have to treat patients as part of your practice. There's no difference in terms of the
psychopharmacology. Now, as far as the promotional gimmicks
and those things that go on, that's very simple, too. I'm on the
Board of Medical Psychology and we have board certified every
one of the medical psychologists that are prescribing. And in the
last couple of weeks we have actually taken away some board certifications from them for various reasons. Not because they committed any error, because, in fact, there's not one case that we can
find where any psychologist that's prescribing has harmed a patient. There have been no lawsuits in a period now of two decades.
But the fact that remains is that we have standards for those board
certifications. And if you're not going to abide by those standards,

then we're taking that board certification away. Again, codify it in the statute. That's the best way of doing it. Why? Number one, if you violate a statute, then at least something can be done.

One of the things that David Healy talked about this morning was how lawyers might approach this. Lawyers are certainly getting involved in this. Last week, I met with the Trial Lawyers Association about the issue of the liability of physicians and what they should be doing about it. And they said, you know, we agree with you. They knew about the things that I had written and what we're talking about with the campaign. They said we will tell you what our problem is. We have been suing these people for years. You just don't know about it. And the reason why you don't know about it is because, as soon as we file a lawsuit, they settle and then they force the parties to sign a nondisclosure agreement. And the problem lies not with the lawyers because the truth is the lawyers do not really want to sign that. It is the patients who agree to sign because that's how they get paid off. So even from a legal perspective—and I can tell you that there's plenty of legal reasoning right now—I don't think that a lot of these physicians realize the potential liability they have because the quantity of these suits is not disclosed. They cannot blame the drug companies for their writing a script for an ineffective drug. The drug companies are immune from that. The drug companies are only on the hook if they put out a drug that is contaminated or defective. Do you realize that if thalidomide were introduced today, we would probably have maybe 200,000 babies without arms and legs? The reason why we only had seventeen cases in the United States in the later part of the 1950s and early part of the '60s with thalidomide is because there was a courageous commissioner on the FDA who forced them to take it off the market. Where David practices in Europe, that's where they had all the cases with these thalidomide babies, because the Europeans did not take it off the market. Today, that would be totally reversed: In Europe, you would probably find probably none or maybe a few babies that have been affected with thalidomide and we'd have a couple hundred thousand here because we allow physicians to do whatever they want because they have an unlimited license. That is the problem. You have a limited license. I have a limited license. They have an unlimited license.

DR. CUMMINGS (from the audience): I'm compelled to underscore what John and David are talking about. When mental health professionals decide who gets medication or who should get off of medication, and as I described this morning, this is what we found in fifteen years of experience. At American Biodyne, with fifteen years of experience, in fifty states, with twenty-five million enrollees, involving ten thousand psychotherapists, doing millions and millions of episodes, we never had a single malpractice suit, not one, single malpractice suit.

Find me a delivery system of that magnitude that can say, in fifteen years they've never had a malpractice suit. The malpractice suits are out there. My son is general counsel for one of the biggest health organizations in the country, and he underscores what John says: 99% of the lawsuits they settle and the settlement includes a nondisclosure agreement so that the person who sued and settles can never mention that he or she sued. So it sounds as if there are no lawsuits out there. You have no idea the hundreds and thousands of lawsuits that are occurring over mis-prescribing. In contrast, what happened in appropriate prescribing? American Biodyne, with ten thousand mental health professionals extensively and appropriately trained, in fifteen years, with twenty-five million patients, with tens of millions of episodes, there was not a single, solitary lawsuit.

Now, I want to add just one thing. Ever since the 1980s, psychiatrists don't get training in psychotherapy. That was dropped because that's talk therapy. They said that doesn't work. So we had psychiatrists in American Biodyne write the script when a mental health professional referred a patient for it. I was visiting one of our centers, not in Arizona, and I wanted to see one of our psychiatrists. The receptionist said, "Oh, Dr. Cummings, he's with a patient." I thought since he is doing some kind of medical evaluation, he'll be out in a few minutes as the psychotherapist, in referring the patient, had already made the decision as part of the referral. When twenty minutes, had passed I asked the receptionist why he was taking so long. She replied, "Oh, he's doing psychotherapy." I waited until he came out, and I said, "You are not qualified to do psychotherapy because you have never, never been trained in psychotherapy." And he said to me, "I'm a psychiatrist. I can do anything I want." And I said, "Not in my company. You have to agree that this will never happen again." He curtly replied, "I won't." To which as curtly, I said, "You're fired." He sued me. It wasn't even heard by court as his suit was thrown out.

So, colleagues, what John and David are saying, when you are doing behavioral care with a patient and you know your patient, you are for sure not going to prescribe an antidepressant to a pregnant woman. You wouldn't think of doing that. You know your patient.

So, I want to underscore what you guys are saying. I can't agree with you more. And if you could find me a health plan fifteen years, 25 million enrollees, 10,000 therapists without a single lawsuit, I want to meet that company.

DOCTOR CACCAVALE: One thing I would like to add as I know Robert Whitaker is going to be presenting this tomorrow, one would have thought that the expose that Robert has given to us, we would have made some real changes. But, in fact, his revelations haven't really made the changes in mental health practice and certainly not in healthcare. It's a Bible for lawyers, as they have used his book and they've been very effective with it. When I was talking with the trial lawyers, they brought up his name immediately. I mean, we're stuck. You know, we have a real problem here, and trying to find the solution is extremely difficult because, number one, we are the Davids alongside the Goliaths. There's no question about that. So we need to find the hole in the wall into which we can poke our finger, not to plug it, but to make the wall come down, because it's the wall that's the problem.

DOCTOR O'DONOHUE: Before we take questions from the audience, let me ask this one question. Do you see anything in President Obama's health-care reform that would have any positive impact on this? Obama's health-care reform is a big thing and it's a moving target.

DOCTOR CACCAVALE: Well, I mean, calling it reform is the problem because there's not really much of a reform. Now, what's it going to do, it's going to solidify the system even further, because, unfortunately, the healthcare reform bill was worked out in private with the pharmaceuticals and the insurers. And of course they're really big in terms of this medical home model, and that's the big word now. If anything, it's going to solidify the system as it is and make it even more difficult to change.

The positive thing that I see coming out of that healthcare reform is perhaps inadvertent. I was on a team with *Huffington Post* doing an analysis of the Kennedy bill passed several years ago before Ted Kennedy died. Most things that happen with policy are completely opposite of what you would expect. And the one positive thing that I see coming out of healthcare reform is that, when you add 30 million people onto rolls, there will be such a shortage of physicians that people will be forced to pay in order to get healthcare. That is going, in my view, to force a fiduciary responsibility on the healthcare system. Now, fiduciary responsibility is going to be not only to get the appropriate treatment, but also getting it in time and by the right person.

Another positive that I see coming out of the healthcare reform that is certainly not part of their thinking that went into it. I do believe that fee-for-service will be coming back. And the reason why I think fee-for-service will be coming back is because you cannot add those many millions of people on the rolls without creating a logjam. And when you create a logjam and you create that waiting list that's certainly going to be there, and there are people who are going to be willing to pay for that treatment and getting it when they need it. So I believe that that's going to be the effect, that's going to make some changes there.

The last positive change that I see coming with the health-care reform is that mental health parity that has always been a lot of words and has actually worked to the opposite for mental health, might inadvertently work and not be just a lot of words as in past parity legislation. The mental health parity that is built into the affordable healthcare reform right now allows patients to actually go to almost any provider on an emergency basis. You can go out of network. And so I think that what we tried to do for many years in many states was to try to get any willing provider provisions and statutes, and that has failed. I think that that's one of the things that we'll be seeing is that patients, because of these long waiting lists and the fact that they're forced to pay, will create different runs on the system that could be very positive.

DOCTOR ANTONUCCIO: Just two quick comments on that. I think one good thing that is in the health-care reform bill is where we target some incentives for preventive care. This could be helpful and useful in reducing costs in the long run. We'll see. The mental health parity could in theory be a good thing, but my worry is that it will be parity in terms of, you know, the mental health patient will get as many drugs as the medical patient. So my worry about parity is that it will evolve into really medical treatment parity and not much of what we offer. So we'll see how it evolves.

DR. O'DONOHUE: Okay. Now, we solicit questions from the audience.

AUDIENCE SPEAKER ONE: Well, thanks a lot for taking on these difficult issues. It's really important!

I'm from New Mexico, which, as you know, is the very first state to acquire prescribing privileges, and I just want to say something to the contingencies that Dr. Antonuccio mentioned. In my experience, and this is strictly just based on the colleagues that I know throughout the state, particularly in my local area, that contingency has exactly happened. They've become the de facto psychiatrists in the worst sense of the word. Every prescribing psychologist that I know has fallen into this contingency of doing only medications, only prescriptions, and so now we have to create a whole new tier, particularly in integrated behavioral healthcare in these medical settings, that the psychologist could have done or would have done at one point but they've gotten sucked right into the trap of prescribing. So your idea of standards or statutes may be a solution. But in the reality, at least where I see it coming from, those contingencies and the drives toward medication prescription as being the primary thing they do is what's happened. And, you know, I'd love to see other comparable data or the kinds of things about that.

The other thing that I wanted to say, and it capitalizes on something that Dr. Cummings said and has been saying ever since we have been part of the DBH program, and that is that there's a part of me that says some of your discussion is less relevant now than it might have been or will be less relevant in the future because it's not going to be physicians that we have to worry about endorsing psychotherapy, it's going to be nurse practitioners. I don't see anything about what we're doing to help educate them or partner with them to encourage integrated behavioral care in the behavioral intervention sense. So what do you say about either of them?

DOCTOR ANTONUCCIO: I want to just make one comment about the contingencies. There is a psychiatric nurse I work with at the V.A. in Reno who was a cognitive therapist, and she did that for years, but she wanted to sort of broaden her base and ensure some job security in an environment where it looked like they might be shrinking the staff. So she got the privilege to prescribe psychiatric drugs. And then, unfortunately because she wanted to keep doing therapy, her job became just prescribing pills. So with this one individual, I saw this contingency play out in her career, and she's not happy with the outcome because she's not getting to do what she really wanted to do. That's one case example. But we see this happening at other places too.

DOCTOR CACCAVALE: You know, I would agree as I'm not talking about supporting prescriptive authority with the present prescribing model. That's the point. If we're not going to change the model, then there's no need to add another level of prescribers. And I can tell you that, having been involved with the New Mexico people, and I know most of them too, the problem in New Mexico is that it is the first state to get prescription authority for psychologists. But it was also because of the APA that put out their model legislation, which was defective in the first place. It was not only defective in terms of what they wanted in the legislation, which really was to make them prescribers; it was what was taking place with psychiatrists. At the time that's who they saw as the competitor, psychiatrists, not family practitioners.

And I was part of that debate too. And I had the same position then as I have now, and that is, what is a prescribing psychologist? And their position was, well, we cannot answer that. We don't have to answer that now. Let's wait until everybody's prescribing and then we can define who they are. This was the kind of thinking. Now it is real clear that if you have the present system just being duplicated by clinical psychologists, family practitioners are very glad to hand them off to write the script and take the responsibility, so there's no changes. And then the psychologist would be, as I said in my presentation, an addition to a flawed system. We're just as trapped as regards integrated care, which sounds really good and it certainly should be a goal. But, remember, when you have integrated care, you're also tying yourself to that medical model. I mean, that's one of the things that you have to fight about. We're going to have to resolve that. And if we don't have any good solutions to that in integrated care, we have not solved the problem. That's why I say, if you want to have integrated care, it better be by a mental health professional who can also prescribe because the ability to prescribe is the ability to say no, I'm not going to do that. Otherwise, you're trapped. All you're doing then is writing the script that the family practitioner would have been writing.

And so I understand what's going on in New Mexico. In Louisiana, it's even worse. We have to make sure that those states that were the first states, they're not the model.

DOCTOR O'DONOHUE: Okay. What's the next question?

AUDIENCE SPEAKER TWO: Hi. Thank you for answering our questions. I'm a clinical psychologist, and I worked with physicians in Medicare in nursing homes as part of an integrated team. It seems from my observations with both the nurse practitioners and the medical doctors, that they would often lose perspective, that there was such a reactive environment in skilled nursing facilities that they lose perspective of what is the most ethical thing to do or what is the most even the most effective thing to do. Instead, in this reactive environment, well, what is it I can do now that will most immediately help to calm the situation and to mask the symptoms? It seems that, even though these things that you're saying are true and are based in real science, the ethical, moral piece that I think that a lot of medical doctors will go to school wholeheartedly believing in, once they get into the actual practice, they lose that perspective. And the other part of that is that it's just not profitable in our system today. That's been my observations that to actually take time to make those more ethical decisions isn't profitable. It's much easier just to write a prescription and that takes care of it. And that takes care of their responsibility and covers them, covers their liability as well. So I guess I'm kind of asking a big question, but I'm really wondering about how the ethics and the standards of good science, good treatment, effective treatment that you're talking about can be restored and be profitable. Is that a good-enough question or do you want me to try to make it more specific?

DR. ANTONUCCIO: All right. Yes, and we're going to agree on this one. The first-do-no-harm approach is what do we consider the ethical standard that we should shoot for? Unfortunately, the way psychiatry has evolved, it is a practice of "a pill for every ill," is how I've been phrasing it, that there's a pill for the depression, a pill for the anxiety; there's a pill for the sleep issue. I can tell you from having looked at the literature on combining psychotropics, we could not find any studies that examined more than two psychiatric drugs at a time in a randomized controlled trial. We couldn't find them. So they don't exist. So we have no science to guide us in terms of safety and ethics. So if you want science and the evidence or the data to be your guide and a first-do-no-harm approach be your guide, it differs from average way it's practiced.

DR. CACCAVALE: But I think she's asking in part, can you practice ethically and also survive and make a profit?

AUDIENCE SPEAKER TWO: Yeah.

DR. CACCAVALE: It depends on how you define profit when you really get down to it. If you look at profit as being part of the whole health-care system, there's no question that the ethical practice would actually reduce cost. That's clear. If you're looking at it from the individual practitioner's perspective, that's another issue. If you were a prescribing psychologist, you'd have a waiting list. There would be so much volume, not so much because you're able to prescribe a drug or someone's looking for it, but the fact that you were a full-service provider, and in practicing ethically, it would be no different than it is right now. Most of you who are practicing must have a good reputation; otherwise, you wouldn't get a second patient. One of the hallmarks, I think, that differentiates us from medicine—and maybe I'm wrong about that because I'm being chauvinistic—is that we do enforce ethics on ourselves as psychologists from day one.

Unfortunately, I think a lot of that is being questioned even today, because everyone is worried about how we're going to make the buck because we have a supply-and-demand problem.

AUDIENCE SPEAKER TWO: Well, we've got to pay back our loans.

DR. CACCAVALE: Yeah, you have to pay back loans. It is really crazy when you think about it, that someone has to go to a school and get $150,000 in debt and then make $40,000 a year to repay it. Something's wrong there. I think where your ethical issue really belongs is, why are professional schools training you under those circumstances and under those conditions?

However, the short answer is yes, you can practice ethically and make a profit. Otherwise, we're standing things on their head by saying the best way to make some money is to be unethical. And that's not acceptable.

DR. ANTONUCCIO: Right and I will agree with you that you can have an ethical practice that's profitable if the patients are demanding it and want it, but they have to be educated that they are getting the best kind of treatment that is effective. If they are educated by the direct-to-consumer ads that when they have this ill, they need this pill, then they're going to find a doctor who's going to practice that way. I would not want to go to a doctor who's just going to tell me to do some breathing exercises when this anxiolytic in the ad is really going to help me sleep. Right now the patients are being educated by the drug industry. And so that's a potential roadblock to the ethical practice leading to a profitable practice.

DR. CACCAVALE: I would just add one thing. I've had patients over the years that have had very severe injuries, such as a persistently painful crushed foot that doesn't seem to get better. There is no control over it, and the patient is in constant pain. I've had at least twelve such patients who came to me and said, "My orthopedist said that if you give the okay, he'll amputate my foot." And I respond, "okay, for what?"

The response that if I say the patient is psychologically able to handle this, then the surgeon will do the amputation with the expectation there will be no more pain. I reply that I'm not going to sign that because, number one, it's a lie. You are likely to have more pain. And I explain about phantom pain and other things that might be sequels.

Providers need to have responsibility. That's the key here. The same way you write your name on a script, or you don't have to write your name on a script. That's why I'm not letting these physicians off the hook, not because I do not like physicians, as that's not an issue. It has nothing to do with hurt feelings; it has nothing to do with liking or disliking; it has nothing to do with personal relationships. Rather, it has to do with our need to have responsibility. Physicians cannot keep blaming the drug companies for advertising to consumers, because they are not compelled to write the script. They don't have to succumb to drug company reps who offer them trips to Hawaii. They don't have to go to Hawaii.

The analogy is that of politicians all day long complain that they can't do their job because the lobbyists are pumping too much money into their pockets and they just can't stop taking it. I mean, that's ridiculous. Are we not adults? Let's get real here. Physicians need to take responsibility for what they know. But they also need to take responsibility for what they don't know. If we have to have that responsibility, so would they. I just have a much more hardnosed approach about this because I identify them as the problem.

AUDIENCE SPEAKER THREE: There were a couple of slides shown earlier regarding the fact that a combination of treatments was most effective; that is, a combination of medication and cognitive therapy. I think there are a fair amount of studies that show that. To some degree, it sounds like we're making a false dichotomy here in terms of either/or, when maybe we should be looking at both.

And, also, back to your comments about what treatments are appropriate and under what conditions. There may be some conditions that need both medication and therapy, as a matter of fact, quite a few, rather than sort of parceling them out as separate. Maybe we need to look at how do the two go together. I would also guess that if we combine therapy with medication, we would be using less medication, which will get to the polypharm problem. So I'd like your comments on that.

DR ANTONUCCIO: The TAS study showed, on a global scale, the combination treatment did seem to have a better outcome. But on the specific depression scales, that wasn't true. In the follow-up that just wasn't true. And, in fact, the vast majority of depression studies don't show combination treatment to be better than psychotherapy alone, although a significant plurality of studies do show the combination to be better than drugs alone. So my message to you would be that psychotherapy, and particularly cognitive behavioral treatments, and interpersonal therapy, are effective stand-alone treatments in comparison to the drugs or the combination. So in terms of depression, at least, that's my reading of my summary of it.

DOCTOR O'DONOHUE: I see that David has a question, too.

DOCTOR HEALY (from the audience): Just quickly: You guys are actually both on the same side in some respects. You're both taking a shower approach rather than a bidet approach. You think you're taking a bidet approach. But a little bit of the problem I've got is: I've heard John say a few times now, if you're going to get the drugs, you want the expert there to do it for you.

The problem is, the expert hasn't got any more access to the data than the primary care physician or the nurse would have. In the U.K. we've had a lot more primary care prescribing than you guys have here. We've got less polypharmacy than you have. It's not clear to me that in the U.S., if you have experts, whether they be clinical psychologists or medical specialists that it's going to improve the system. I mean, we're all on the same side. You know, we recognize there's a problem. The repeated recourse we have is to have experts to solve the problem for us, and I think we need to turn a little bit more to patients.

On the expert front, one other note is something John brings out a little bit on the conflicts-of-interest front. What I repeatedly say to people on that is that you don't want to actually depend on me to be a saint. You don't want to actually depend on me to have no links to drug companies or whatever or to be morally good.

Talking about experts is a little bit the same kind of thing. I don't think we should be in the business of having a system that depends on experts, because if it goes wrong, we want greater expertise. We want more and more conflicting interests to be declared. And this isn't the answer to the problem. The answer to the problem is access to the data.

DOCTOR HEALY (still from the audience, but concluding): I throw this open to both of you.

DOCTOR ANTONUCCIO: I would say access to the data is the key. I think we want patients to be in charge of their own care. I think we are consultants more than we are treatment providers per se. And I know that when it comes to my medical care, I want to be the captain of my ship and I want my patients to feel the same way and they ultimately make the decision. Now, they do need information if they are to make informed decisions, and as you pointed out in your wonderful writing, the literature that we rely on is distorted. And that's not a good resource and it's written by the so-called experts. So how we get access to those data? One thing we proposed is that it be required by all higher beings that the data be accessible to all patients. And you can tell from Turner's work that a lot of these patients who participate in these studies not only don't have access to data but the data they produce nobody has access to. So how we solve that is the challenge.

DOCTOR CACCAVALE: A couple of things I would like to say, David, are, first, that even without the data, I know that these drugs can't work. That's the first thing. I mean, the whole chemical imbalance issue, you've gone through that. If you have any kind of training whatsoever, you can understand that it cannot work that way. So if it cannot work that way and you're telling me this is the way it works, that's the first red flag that I have.

The second thing is that obviously it is not only a data problem, because you have the data. David has the data. I have the data. This is what we've been talking about all day today. We're telling them about the data. So it's not a lack of data and it's really not even so much a lack of access when you really get down to it, because if you go to Google and you Google these things, you get a million stories about these drugs. People have access today to information that they never had before.

The problem, again, is that we have to take responsibility as providers. And I'm not willing, you know, to say these poor physicians or the poor psychologists or the poor anybody, they don't have access to data and so therefore that's why they're doing these things even though these things are harmful.

When I speak with physicians, I seem to get answers from them, and they seem to understand. The thing is that many of them feel that if they don't give that script to that patient, that patient's going to feel that they went to that visit for nothing at all. They're not being a doctor. So they have to do something.

They also feel, as you know as a trained physician yourself, you deal with symptoms. Oh, you can't sleep. I'll give you something for sleep. You're not eating? I'll give you something for eating. It's symptom-based.

We also have a problem with the issue of diagnosis and what that really means, and we haven't even talked about that today. So I agree with what you say, but I as I said before, I was never so much against medications until I started training in them. All of a sudden things became very clear.

AUDIENCE SPEAKER FOUR: I think we all agree with the need to inform the system of what's going on, but I'm wondering why we're making villains of the physicians in the process. It seems like we really need to have them on our side because the physicians are the ones that we're working directly with.

In reality, it seems to me, that the health insurance companies are the ones that make the rules. They're the ones that the physicians look to for the rules in what they're going to do. Why aren't they the focus of this campaign?

DOCTOR CACCAVALE: The physician, again, is the person that's making the decision, both legally and clinically. That's the reason. We understand why insurers, for example, would rather pay for a psychotropic drug as opposed to a course of psychotherapy. We understand why the pharmaceuticals would rather the treatment of choice be a pill.

But let me ask you another question. We have a drug policy. People who take the drug are getting treatment. People who sell the drug and distribute the drug get the penalty. Why is that different with physicians? And as far as getting them on our side, this is not an anti-physician campaign. This is an issue of what should be the appropriate treatment by the appropriate person at the appropriate time. This has nothing to do with personalities.

Now, if the physicians were not in this loop, then we would not be talking about physicians. We would be talking about insurers and we would be talking about the pharmaceuticals. But if you take a look at the system, the physicians have control over the treatment. If the physician turned around and said: I'm sorry but, you know, the treatment of choice for this particular patient, based on the data, is that I'm going to send them out to a behavioral health specialist. Then I'll take a look and if I see nothing is happening over there, then I'll have this patient come back and we'll see what we can do. That would be one thing. But that's not what's taking place. And so, if anything, what we should be doing is we should be looking out for the patient's interests, not the physician's interest, not our interest, but the patient's interests. That's this Patients' Bill of Rights. That's this guy here. That's what David Healy is saying also. It would be great if we could get them on our side, but unfortunately we're not even speaking in the same language with physicians on this issue.

I had major physician associations tell me that we cannot sign on to your bill because it has the word "collaboration" in it. When I ask what's wrong with the word "collaboration", the response is that it assumes that we have less control over their treatment. The so-called patient-centered model is a lot of talk. If you look at the medical home model, that reveals what they're talking about. What is the medical home model really? It is family physician over here and everybody else below the family physician. The problem that we have is, again, that the drug companies can put out all the drugs they want, but they're not the ones who can prescribe it. The drug companies can get a penalty for trying to market off-label drugs, but the physician doesn't get a penalty for writing it. So, I mean, the physicians are definitely in the problem loop. They're there, and there's no way that they can be taken out of it. And, again, it's not a personality issue. It's not a liking issue. It's the fact that this is the way the system is. And the same way that we've gone after psychiatry for the kinds of issues and kinds of practices that they've engaged in, how can we not involve the people that are writing 85% of the scripts on these same medications?

DOCTOR O'DONOHUE: David, did you have a comment?

DOCTOR ANTONUCCIO: I have just one comment about it. I'm hoping that in the Patient Bill of Rights we did not put language in there to demonize the prescribers. In fact, the idea is to empower the patients and for the patients to say they want a physician who prescribes according to these principles.

What I actually hope would also happen, but it may not, is that some physicians' group would say they like these like principles enough to join a group that supports prescribing according to these principles. There's the hope that it might even be attractive to some prescribers. My concern comes partly from my own clinical experience. When I have a patient who is suffering side effects from medications, it has never worked for me to call up the doctor and say that I think this patient might be suffering some side effects. Invariably the doctor feels defensive and I get a negative response. Whereas, if the patient says, you know, Doctor, I'd like your help coming off this medicine, or I'd like your help in dealing with the side effect that I'm experiencing, would then not patients be more likely to have a good outcome?

So I don't want to, nor do I intend to, have the Bill of Rights demonize physicians' prescribing practices or the physicians themselves. The idea is to empower the patients so they can ask for the kind of treatment that is ethical, safe, and effective.

DOCTOR CACCAVALE: I don't like your word "demonize."

DOCTOR ANTONUCCIO: Right. Well, I'm....

DOCTOR CACCAVALE: That's an inappropriate word.

DOCTOR ANTONUCCIO: I think that's what she was asking.

DOCTOR CACCAVALE: No, I'm talking about not demonizing physicians.

DOCTOR ANTONUCCIO: Well, I'm not suggesting you are. But I was responding to her question.

AUDIENCE SPEAKER FIVE: This sort of goes off of what you're talking about, but I was wondering about the general stigma that the general public has about mental illness. Only 1% of mentally ill challenged people commit a hideous crime, yet that's what hits the news. And actually there's a provider in this area that just sent out a memo regarding their job performance in public safety. So do you think if we educated the general public more on mental illness that it could help the cause any?

DOCTOR ANTONUCCIO: So what you're saying is that a small percentage of mentally ill patients engage in criminal behavior? Is that what you're saying?

AUDIENCE SPEAKER FIVE: Yes, that's what I've been told.

DOCTOR ANTONUCCIO: And yet it's been sensationalized when it does happen.

AUDIENCE SPEAKER: Yeah.

DOCTOR ANTONUCCIO: And so the mental health community gets blamed? Am I understanding your question right? Part of your question, I think, seems to be also including a solution, which I think is right; that of educating people how rare this is and how it's the exception. But you know the way our media works, that may get obscured by the big story.

AUDIENCE SPEAKER FIVE: So you feel educating the general public wouldn't play a huge part in all this.

DOCTOR ANTONUCCIO: I think that would be a good first step.

AUDIENCE SPEAKER FIVE: In changing the system?

DR. ANTONUCCIO: I think that would be an important step, yes.

AUDIENCE SPEAKER SIX: As a primary care provider, I can tell you from where some of these issues arise. I work in a small rural clinic right now, but I did five-and-a-half years at Mayo Clinic in Rochester, Minnesota. And one thing that I noticed with new nurse practitioners and residents and so on is that they understand what they can do, but they don't know what they should do. And I'll give you an example of that.

About two weeks ago, I got a phone call from a cardiologist who said that he saw my patient in the clinic and she's refusing to take her statin. And you need to get her to take her statin. I said that theoretically she should take a statin, but she's 88 years old. I'm not going to trash her liver. If she hasn't had a heart attack by now, she's not going to have a heart attack.

So it's things like that. Let's order an echocardiogram on this lady. But what are we going to do with those results? It's not going to change our outcome, so on and so forth. So they go through their textbook and they understand what they can do, but they don't know what they should do. They don't know when to stop and they don't know when to turn it off. And I think part of it is fear. You know, like you were talking about the docs that got sacked. And I worry about that too because I try to get as many patients as I can off as many medications as I can. But I do worry that someone is going to do a chart review and say, well, you know, you took this patient off her statin. Why did you do that? You know, it's kind of a fear situation, too.

So until we educate the residents and educate the medical community to say, look, it's okay to be off these medications, it's okay to let the patient choose, it's not going to change.

DR. ANTONUCCIO: Right. And I would say, you're not really taking your patient off. Your patient is making that choice. To me, that would be the defense, that patients have a right to choose their treatment intervention.

AUDIENCE SPEAKER SIX: What I find interesting is being placed as a physician in the position where you're promoting health and having to fear that you'll get sacked for promoting health. Because, quite frankly, I don't know who you are, but I want your card, because if I'm going to be treated, I'd rather be treated by you.

DOCTOR ANTONUCCIO: Me too.

DOCTOR CACCAVALE: So I'll sign on right now. And I think you illustrate exactly what we're talking about, that you as a physician take a personal responsibility and act that way. And if you can do it, I don't see why we're giving a pass to others.

DOCTOR ANTONUCCIO: Can you start a group of physicians who practice like that so people can go to it. The public needs to know that there can be careful, conservative treatment? Are there organizations like that?

DOCTOR CACCAVALE: There is. In fact, there's a whole group of physicians called "Lifestyle Medicine Practitioners," and that's exactly what they do. They don't run to statins, for example, with cardiac problems. The first thing they look at is diet and exercise and those kinds of things. But they've been shut out of primary care for the most part because a lot of primary care physicians or family physicians don't really see that as a practice because they can't make money because they can't see people in two minutes. They have to work, you know, with a limited time with people.

Also, the reimbursement schedules are not set out for them to be practicing the way they do. The economic incentives are in the wrong direction, or what economists call "perverse incentives." No matter how one wants to look at it, that's the proximate cause of our problem. All these other issues may also be contributing. But let's face it. You know, when you're trying to find a solution, but you have a million causes, it becomes almost impossible. You have to kind of prioritize what it is that you can do and what is it that you cannot do. And I just think that education is always something that we need to be doing and that's extremely important. All I know is, however, as a practitioner, when people come in, somehow their intellectual abilities just go out the window. It is as if they are saying, "I just need to be taken care of." That's just the way it is. And that makes things a little bit more difficult.

On our website truthindrugs.com, if you go there, last week we put out a sheet for parents to bring to their physician with the questions that they should be asking their physician if a physician wants to medicate their kids. One of the things that we didn't even talk about today is the absolute disgrace of what we're doing with children with ADHD, just giving them psycho-stimulants. I mean, we can go on and on and on and on. Talking tomorrow will be Dr. Casciani who's an expert with seniors. What are we doing with seniors? We passed a prescription bill to give them more drugs that they don't need.

David Healy was showing you, as was David here, what happens when you take people off medications. They actually get better. So, this is an immense problem and we need to find a way. And what I'm suggesting to you is that we need to address the family physicians and the primary care physicians who are practicing not like this lady in the back. They're the low-hanging fruit and they're the ones that we need to grab because they're there and they're the easiest ones because she's right: It is fear. And when they start to see that there's a real fear in the liability that they have, I assure you that those changes will take place a lot faster than educating the whole population.

AUDIENCE SPEAKER SEVEN: Yes, sir. Earlier somebody had brought up the public education component of what you're doing, and I'm reminded by looking at your ad, who did you design that ad for?

DOCTOR CACCAVALE: That ad was actually designed for the public.

AUDIENCE SPEAKER SEVEN: It doesn't look like it's designed for a consumer. It looks like a cigarette warning label that has all those things have been ignored for how many years now? I mean, I'm just kind of putting that out to you, who's it really targeted to?

DOCTOR CACCAVALE: That's who it was designed for and, again, everything that we have on there comes from the FDA and it's a grabber. That's what it's about.

AUDIENCE SPEAKER SEVEN: Have you ever considered hiring an actual design firm to design your ad instead of going by the FDA?

DOCTOR CACCAVALE: In fact, that's what we did. It was a media consultant who did it. In fact, it was a media consultant who is very well known for his political ads. I mean, that's politics up there.

AUDIENCE SPEAKER SEVEN: Ah, maybe that's the problem.

DOCTOR CACCAVALE: Well, it's not the problem. The problem is that if you look at it as a mental health professional, you're going to have one reaction to that.

AUDIENCE SPEAKER SEVEN: No, I understand that. I'm living proof about everything you're saying about drugs and everything. I mean, I've been a consumer for twenty years and I take no medications. I've been very well off. But when I see that ad and everything you're trying to do, it almost seems like you're fighting with each other instead of trying to really inform the public. Do you think it's any coincidence that peer recovery is such a movement in this country and New Zealand? And guess what? We're the two countries in the world that allow direct marketing to consumers. I think that's a mistake. That's all I've got.

DOCTOR CACCAVALE: Well, it's not and that's why we're against direct marketing to consumers.

AUDIENCE SPEAKER EIGHT: You referred a little bit earlier to the diagnosis issue, and I was just wondering if you could expand on that a little bit, because it seems to me that that's kind of the elephant in the room today. What drives a lot of the prescribing is the idea that we have diseases here that need to be treated in a medical way, using the medical model. And so, you know, we have a whole DSM system that's designed around that idea. So isn't that really sort of the core of the problem? That is, how we conceptualize these behavioral conditions as diseases? I was just wondering about your thoughts on that.

DOCTOR CACCAVALE: Yeah, I think both of us would probably again agree on this completely. I mean, look how the DSMs have been designed, as well as the one that's coming out next year or two years from now. DSM-5 is going to be probably one of the biggest jokes that you're ever going to see. Clearly! If you develop a system to where the treatment is drugs and you're medicalizing that through the DSM. Don't forget who publishes the DSM. It's owned and published by the American Psychiatric Association. So, are there things in the DSM that are pretty ridiculous and stupid? Are there things in the DSM that point towards medicalization? Absolutely! So the problem is that we have a diagnostic category that's based on probably a lot of flimsy concepts that are the same way some of these medications are. But they're headed to that direction.

So what is it that you do about it? Well, the truth is that in my practice, I didn't use the DSM much at all. I used the ICD. I don't know when the last time I ever bought a DSM. To me it's a lot of foolishness. I think we could all agree on the fact that, you maybe we shouldn't have a category called "depression." Maybe we should just have something called "a mood disorder" and then, you know, describe what those kinds of things are. But that's what I said. If you're going to be looking at psychotherapy, then we should have it related to something that's a condition, a real condition. And we don't have that now.

DOCTOR ANTONUCCIO: And one comment on this: The DSM is constructed so that of course the person can have multiple diagnoses, and if you take the disease model, you give a pill for each separate entity as if they're somehow unrelated. But it turns out, you don't need to have multiple diagnoses to get multiple pills. You can get a pill for every symptom within one category. So our system is not working well.

AUDIENCE SPEAKER EIGHT: A very good point that you make.

AUDIENCE SPEAKER NINE: Thank you. Well, first of all, I want to say that I found the advertising fantastic, in my opinion. And I also wanted to ask, I work in the field of substance abuse and most of the people I work with come and ask me in a very open and honest and maybe genuine way, what's the big difference between street drugs and the psychoactive substances? And before, at least until today, maybe I used to be lying to these people, to my people, saying, the big difference is that the psycho-active substances that your doctor prescribes, they are supposed to heal, whereas the other ones, well, they just provide a momentary fix. So I don't really know as of tomorrow what to tell my people. What do you suggest I say?

DOCTOR ANTONUCCIO: What a great question. And you know what? I don't know. I want to think that one through before I even answer. I mean, maybe Healy or you or somebody else has something, but that's a thought-provoking question that I want to think on overnight, actually.

DOCTOR CACCAVALE: It is a great question and a more difficult is, what are you trying to achieve with the patient? If you look at addiction medicine, a lot of the addiction today is because people are being addicted by prescription meds. I mean, because rather than street drugs you're too often looking at OxyContin, Vicodin, Soma, and Xanax. The most difficult patient I ever had to treat was the patient who was prescribed Lorazepam over ten years ago and never got off of it. I was never able to get my patient off of it, either. And so the difference between these drugs is that one is being written and obtained legally and one is not.

But, in fact, they're doing the same thing. So when you're looking at narcotics, I think the question is a lot easier. When you're looking at it compared to some of these other classes of drugs, I, like David, would have to really think about that. And the reason why I'd have to think about that is because there are those 9% to 15% of patients who may benefit from some of these drugs. Our problem is that, as long as we're wholesale writing prescriptions and we're not dealing with the data, then we're not going to know which ones they are.

DOCTOR O'DONOHUE : Okay, with that we have to close. Thank you very much.

Applause.

Chapter 6

# Anatomy of an Epidemic: History, Science, and the Case Against Psychiatric Drugs

*Robert Whitaker*
*(Edited version of presentation published by permission)*

Yesterday, when listening to those great talks, I thought, they are hard talks to follow they were so good. It made me think of how extraordinarily important this subject is. If you look at how the use of psychiatric drugs is changing our society, of which you heard a lot about yesterday, it is vitally important. For example, we heard from David Healy that 15% of all mothers when they give birth are on antidepressants. So one out of every six children is now being born to a mother who has been taking an antidepressant while she was pregnant. And if you look at those data, there is some question about how that will affect that child's development and later life. So it's a big question. As you know, we are now medicating two year-olds, five year-olds, and so on. I can't even figure out what percent of American children really are medicated today, but I think it's over 10%. So that's a big number. I recently was speaking at an association of college counselors in the Northeast. These college counselors work for liberal arts schools, so maybe this number is too high because I'm picking a certain type of population. They say now that 28% of their incoming freshmen have a prescription for a psychotropic drug, showing the pervasiveness of this change in our society. Obviously, if you look at the usage in our society as a whole in adults, this medical model, this whole revolution has sort of changed our philosophy of being and our sense of how resilient we might be in the face of certain crises. We get the ads directed to consumers that make you think you're supposed to be happy all the time. And then of course we also heard about the elderly on these drugs as well. So I came away yesterday thinking anew about how pervasive and how profound this subject is because it is changing us as a people. And we really want to know, as it's changing childhood and how we raise our children, is it working for us?

I heard yesterday from David that so much of the information flow that we are given, upon which we to try to base our answers, is corrupt. So we can't even trust the scientific journals to really help us understand a lot about the effects of these drugs. In David Healy's talk, you can't trust the data because it is being spun. You even have questions about the outcome measures. There are a lot of questions in terms of the data out there that's guiding us.

And then we had the second question: Even if the data were good, would the doctors, would the medical community, change their prescribing habits to be consistent with those data? And that's the last two talks we've had. So I'm saying to you as psychologists and other professionals, you are entering a very, very, very, very profound arena of care and trying to sift through the information to figure out what is known and what is not known is very difficult. What I did in *Anatomy of an Epidemic* in essence was to try to put it in a big-picture way, "Is this paradigm of care that we've adopted working for us?" And one of the things I think I did in *Anatomy of an Epidemic,* which hadn't really been done before, is really look at how it's shaping long-term outcomes. So that's new, because even the data you heard yesterday from David is really focused on trials that are of short term. So one of the things to consider is the perspective of long-term outcomes.

The common wisdom, of course, in the history of psychiatry is that it's working great, because Thorazine, when it arrived into asylum medicine in 1955, it kicked off a psychopharmacological revolution. And you can read quotes like that from Edward Shorter (1997) in a book called *The History Psychiatry.* He says that the introduction of Thorazine into asylum medicine in 1955 "initiated a revolution in psychiatry comparable to the introduction of penicillin in general medicine." So that's the story of this great leap forward, and if you read psychiatry texts, they often refer to the psychopharmacological revolution. And listen to the language: Thorazine arrives as the first of the antipsychotics, putting it in the frame of a reference of as antibiotics (e.g., penicillin) for bacterial diseases. And if that were so, it would be a great leap forward, as one of the greatest leaps forward in all of medical history was the discovery of the antibiotics. So how does this story of the psychopharmacological revolution go? We get antipsychotics. We get antidepressants. We get anti-anxiety agents. Those are the first generation drugs. And then beginning in 1987, we get Prozac. It actually arrives on the market in 1988. That, of course, is an SSRI. This is the first of the second generation drugs that is said to be so much safer and more effective than the old drug. Then we get the atypical antipsychotics, and so on. We are told that these drugs fix chemical imbalances in the brain. That becomes popularized with Prozac. If that's true, that is also a story of progress, because that means you've identified the pathology and now you have a drug that is fixing that pathology. It's a specific remedy (see Silverman, 1968; U.S. Social Security Administration Reports, 2007).

We were also told that these drugs are like insulin for diabetes. And that, obviously, is a rationale for long-term use as well. If you have this consistent chemical imbalance, you need to take the drugs for life. And this is the story that was told to us as a story of medical progress. It's really a story that of medical progress that proceeded in two stages. We got the first generation drugs and then the second generation drugs. And in 1998, David Thatcher, who was the U.S. Surgeon General, issued a 400-page report in which he tells this story of progress. He says that prior to 1955, psychiatry lacked treatments that could prevent people from becoming chronically ill. In other words, the course of mental disorders prior to the arrival of the antipsychotics and antidepressants was a chronic course. That's what he's telling us, that it was a disabling course. And we got these drugs and now no longer do mental disorders run a chronic course, since we now have these enabling drugs. That's the message: that these drugs enable people to go back to work and lead relatively normal lives. So the first step is to put that story under a microscope, which is what I did. I looked at the number of people under government care due to mental illness, sometimes referred to as the disabled mentally ill in research. Okay? So in 1955, the "disabled mentally ill" were taken care of in state and county mental hospitals. And at that time there were about 560,000 people in state and county hospitals. But you need to look at little bit deeper into that number because about 200,000 of those people actually did not have psychiatric ailments. They were there with Alzheimer's, end-stage syphilis, that sort of thing. There were 360,000 people with a psychiatric diagnosis. And if you do the per capita rating, that's a disability rate of around 1 in 480 people. Okay? That's at the start of this revolution.

# Did Mental Disability Change
# after Psychotropics?

Now, generally you think, if you get a very effective treatment, you're going to see the disability rate due to that problem decline, right? That generally is what happens. Or at the very least, you would hope it would stay the same. As you know, we de-institutionalized after that. We decided to move our care of the seriously mentally ill into the community, and what others who have tracked this number of the disabled mentally ill have said is this: Well, you have to look at your SSI (Social Security Insurance) and your SSDI (Social Security Disability Insurance) numbers. Right? You're all familiar with that? So, you look at the people who were declared eligible for those programs due to mental illness in ages 18 to 66. Those are the years that are pertinent.

Doing that, we find that in 1987 there were 1.25 million people on disability due to mental illness. That's a rate around 1 in 180. So in spite of the predictions to contrary, we went from 1 in 480 to 1 in 180 (U.S. Social Security Administration Reports. 2007).

Now, someone might say you're comparing apples to oranges, that you had to be more severely mentally ill to be hospitalized than to be on SSI and SSDI and so it's not a fair comparison. Fortunately, however, since 1987 forward, we're using the same metric. In other words, we are using the SSI and SSDI metric. And 1987 is the year we got Prozac. This is when we got the second-generation drugs, and this is when we really embraced the medical model. For example, we spent around $8 million as a society on psychiatric drugs in 1987. In 2007, it was more than $40 billion, so there was a 50-fold increase in 20 years (Silverman, 1968; U.S. Social Security Reports, 1987-2007).

What happened in the number of disabled mentally ill in that time? It went up to more than 4 million people. So it tripled during that time. And here is another way to look at this rise in the number of disabled mentally ill. In 1955, there were 213 per hundred thousand population, then 543 per hundred thousand in 1987, and then 1315 per hundred thousand in 2007. So you see this extraordinary rise in the number of disabled mentally ill, especially in the Prozac era.

These next data are startling, and I discovered them when I was writing my book, *Anatomy of an Epidemic* (Whitaker, 2010). What I found out was, between 1990 and 2003, according to epidemiological surveys, the prevalence of all mental disorders in the United States stayed the same. In other words, the percentage of the population that was said to be suffering from a mental disorder in 1990 and 2003 was the same. What changed, along with an obvious increase in population, was the number of people treated. The percentage of those treated for the disorder doubled. So I get the numbers, and what do you find? You find that the number of adults (not children) who were treated almost doubled between 1990 and 2003, from 11.16 million to 21.77 million. What is the result? We have more than a doubling of the number of people on disability during this time.

Now, this in itself doesn't prove anything, but I think you start to see this is raising questions. What's going on? Why do we have this rise in disability? I was recently giving a talk in Iceland, so I looked at disability numbers in Iceland. There it went up, too. Iceland also has done some tracking of antidepressant use, and it really starts going up at around 1992 (Thoriacius, 2010). I gave a talk in the United Kingdom where I found the same thing: there was a rise in disability numbers (Moncrieff, 2000). So this raises a question. What's going on?

## The Question of Causation

As many people pointed out, this doesn't show causation. It doesn't show that the drugs are causing this disability, but it does raise two questions that I think we need to ask. First, how do drugs shape the long-term course of major mental disorders? In other words, do they increase the likelihood that you're going to work, increase the likelihood that you're going to be healthy, that sort of thing? Or for some reason, does this paradigm of care in the aggregate worsen long-term outcomes, increase the risk of disability, and increase the risk that you won't be working? Does it increase the risk that you'll end up having chronic symptoms? So I think you can see that's a legitimate question raised by these data.

The second question you have to ask is this: Is it possible that with this paradigm of care you can worsen someone with a milder problem such as a mild bout of depression that in the past would have passed on its own if you hadn't medicated the person? Is it possible that once you put people on an antidepressant, there may be a percentage of people who will have a bad reaction to that drug, such as a manic episode? And then, once they have that manic episode, they're going to move from a depression diagnosis to a bipolar diagnosis? And if that's so, you might have mechanism for creating patients. Do you see what I'm saying? People can come in with a milder problem that maybe would have resolved itself, but now you end up with a person who goes into the bipolar category that often comes with a lot of drugs. So the question is, how do medications shape the long-term course of major mental disorders, and do we have a mechanism for possibly creating mental patients? Those are the two questions I tried to answer in *Anatomy of an Epidemic.*

There are a couple of other things to consider if you dig into the disability numbers. What's driving the adult disability numbers? It's largely the affective disorders; i.e., depression and bipolar. For example, if you were to go back to the early 1990s and survey the people on disability, most would have been there with a psychotic diagnosis. In contrast today in a comparable group from 18 to 26 years, more than half have an affective disorder diagnosis: anxiety, depression, bipolar. So we wonder: where are all these affective disorders coming from? Why is this happening?

A second little thing to consider is the scope of this epidemic. Consider that 850 adults per day are going on disability in the United States each of 365 days a year.

## What Is Happening to our Children?

Now, the other very important question is: what's happening to the kids that we really began medicating in the early 1990s? In 1987, the start of this change, there were 16,200 children in the United States 0 to 18 on SSI due to mental illness. Today there are more than six hundred thousand. So that's a 35-fold increase. The number of kids going on disability now per year is about one hundred thousand, so that's about 250 children per day. And when they reach eighteen, if you track these children on medication, they're going right on to adult disability. So you see this pathway has opened up in our society where kids get diagnosed, treated, and then face the life of a mental patient stretching out ahead of them. So you definitely want to figure out what's going on there as well. So a lot of similar questions need to be asked about what is happening to our children.

## The Story of the Chemical Imbalance Hypothesis

The first thing I wanted to do in my book was to put the chemical imbalance story under the microscope because that does drive our care. It influences our societal understanding of what's going on, so I wanted to look at how that story arose and what did they find out when they investigated it.

What you find with the chemical imbalance theory of mental disorders that arose in the 1960s, is that it arose from an understanding of how the drugs acted on the brain as opposed to investigations of people so diagnosed. For example, researchers found that the antipsychotics worked by blocking dopamine receptors in the brain. First, how do neurons communicate? There is the presynaptic neuron that releases that neurotransmitter into the synaptic cleft, the very small gap between neurons. Then it binds with receptors on the post-synaptic neuron, and that's how the message gets passed. So what does Thorazine and the other drugs do? They gum up the receptors, specifically about 70% of a particular type of receptor called the D2 receptor. It's like the old key and lock analogy that the molecule fits like the key into the lock, with the receptor being the lock. Basically, what the drugs do is they block the locks, 70% of them. Once that was understood, that you were thwarting dopamine transmission, researchers hypothesized that people with schizophrenia had overactive dopamine systems. So it was an understanding of the drug's mechanism of action that gave rise to that thesis (Hyman, 1996).

The depression story is the same. They came to understand how monoamine oxidase inhibitors, or the tricyclics, work and they theorized the opposite. And just for clarity's sake, the drugs that we really heard this with were the SSRIs and how they work. Well, what happens with an SSRI? Serotonin gets released into that synaptic cleft and then the brain, in order to make that message sharp, has to remove the serotonin from the cleft. It does that in one or two ways: either an enzyme comes along and metabolizes the serotonin in that cleft and that metabolite is carted off as waste, or the serotonin goes back up the re-uptake channels into the presynaptic neuron. What does Prozac or any of these other drugs do? They block the re-uptake channels so the serotonin stays longer in the synaptic cleft. This is an excitatory neurotransmitter, and theoretically it increases serotonergic transmission. So once researchers understood that, they hypothesized that people with depression had low serotonin.

But what happened when researchers investigated to see if people actually had such chemical imbalances? Real quickly: On the schizophrenia side, in order to see whether these patients had overactive dopamine systems, they first wanted to look at whether those presynaptic neurons put out more dopamine than normal as a matter of course. When they looked at that in patients that were not medicated, they found that not to be so. So then researchers thought maybe people with schizophrenia have too many receptors for dopamine. In never medicated people, they did not find that to be so. So those two keys things were not found. These conclusions are from extensive research over a period of years involving a number of reported studies. A more detailed explanation is in Chapter 5 of my book (Whitaker, 2010).

In their investigation of the low serotonin theory of depression, how did researchers begin to investigate? As you will recall, the serotonin is metabolized and a metabolite is carted off to the cerebral spinal fluid. So what researchers did is, they measured the levels of that metabolite in the cerebral spinal fluid, and they figured that would be a gauge of serotonergic activity. Right? Does that make sense? And so they theorized that people with depression should have lower amounts of the metabolites in the cerebral spinal fluid. And back in the 1970s they find that depressed people have sort of a bell curve in terms of the amounts of that metabolite in the cerebral spinal fluid, meaning there's some at the low end, some in the middle, and some at the high end. If they compared that to metabolites in normal people, they basically are the same. So this actually led to the thought, well, we still have that low end of the bell curve. There is that subgroup of depressed patients with low serotonin metabolites. So researchers theorized, well, maybe that's the group that's really going to respond to antidepressants because as we know, not everybody responds. As early as 1983, the NIMH conducted a trial to investigate this. And what did the researchers find? There was no relationship between the metabolite levels of the patients and response to the drug. In other words, those with high metabolite levels were just as likely to respond as those with low metabolite levels. So as early as 1984, the NIMH concluded that elevations or detriments in the functioning of serotonergic systems per se are not likely to be associated with depression. That's three years before Prozac came on the market.

There has been a lot of other research on this, and researchers just don't find, as a matter of course, that people with depression prior to being medicated have low serotonin. For example, you can read the response of molecular psychiatrist Stephen Stahl (2000), in his book *Essential Psychopharmacology*, "There is no convincing evidence that monoamine deficiency accounts for depression; that is, there is no real monoamine deficit." (Note: serotonin is a monoamine.)

I could go through the history of the research for schizophrenia where you find the same sort of thing. For example, Steven Hyman (2002), who as a neuroscientist was a former director of the NIMH and today is Provost of Harvard University, states, "There is no compelling evidence that a lesion in the dopamine system is a primary cause of schizophrenia."

Finally, Kenneth Kendler (2005), co-editor-in-chief of *Psychological Medicine*, stated: "We have hunted for big simple neurochemical explanations for psychiatric disorders and we have not found them."

In spite of what these neuroscientists say, the public believes differently. Recently there was a survey of the American population, and people were asked, what causes depression? 80% of Americans replied that depression is caused by low serotonin. 87% of Americans replied that schizophrenia is caused by a chemical imbalance too, presumably an overactive dopamine system. So I think you're beginning to see a problem here, and that is that we have this societal delusion in that we believe we have found these biological causes for mental disorders. We believe the drugs are fixing that biological abnormality. But they're not, which can be a problem when we try to think about how to use medications judiciously.

## What Do These Drugs Do?

So the next question is, then: Well, what do the drugs do and how does the brain respond to the drugs? So let's just look at the SSRIs. So the SSRIs keep that serotonin in the synaptic cleft longer than normal. Right? They block the re-uptake, and then the brain, being this extraordinarily responsive thing, responds. It has all these feedback loops. So what does the brain do when that serotonin stays in that synaptic cleft longer than normal? It sort of says: Uh-oh. This is a problem. And it tries to compensate for that. So the drug is acting as an accelerator. What happens in response? The presynaptic neuron, at least for a period of time, starts putting out less serotonin. And what happens in the postsynaptic neuron is a decrease in the number of receptors for serotonin. This is called "down regulation." Does it make sense? The postsynaptic neuron is becoming less sensitive to serotonin. And you can see why this might be so. The drug tries to put down the accelerator on serotonergic transmission. The brain responds by putting down the brake.

I'm thinking now about the antipsychotics. What do they do? They block dopamine. Right? It's like putting down the brake. So what does the brain do in response? It tries to put down the accelerator. At least for a time, the presynaptic neurons put out lower dopamine. That compensatory mechanism begins to break down after time. In addition, the postsynaptic neurons increase the density of the D2 receptors by about 50%. That's called "up regulation."

So I think you can see a little bit of a prior here. Prior to taking the medication, people with schizophrenia or depression have no known abnormality. Once they're on the drugs, they do. They will have these different receptor densities.

In 1996, when Steven Hyman was director of the NIMH, he wrote a brilliant paper called *A Paradigm for Understanding Psychotropic Drugs*, and I would suggest all of you may want to read that paper. By the way, I hope that you see what I'm doing here. I'm following the mainstream research as I do this. I'm following what the NIMH found, and what is being announced by the molecular psychiatry docs. Okay? And here's what Hyman said: "These drugs work by perturbing neurotransmitter systems in the brain. In response to that perturbation, the brain undergoes compensatory adaptations in order to maintain its homeostatic equilibrium" [in other words, it's trying to maintain these normal pathways]. And he further says, "At the end of this adaptive process, the brain is operating in a manner that is both qualitatively and quantitatively different than normal." Now, that doesn't tell you anything about whether these medications are going to be useful long term. But it does raise a couple of things. Is this a normalizing paradigm of care? No. In other words, we don't know the pathology, and so the drugs are not fixing something. The drugs in fact are throwing a wrench into normal functioning, and the brain tries to adapt to that wrench and now the brain operates differently. In response to that, maybe someone is going to have different moods, different mood stabilization, whatever it might be. But you can see that's a very different conception of the drug. I think once you have this conception, you can understand why the drugs may have a lot of adverse effects because they're not normalizing agents. That's number one. I think you can understand, too, why withdrawal might be a problem. That is number two. So think about it, once you are on the drug, you actually have an "accelerator–brake" situation going. Antipsychotics act as a brake. The brain has responded by putting down the accelerator. Now let's take away the brake. You might have some real imbalance there, so to speak.

Finally, someone asked yesterday, "What is the difference between illicit drugs and licit drugs?" Well, Steven Hyman actually addresses that in his paper. It's pretty funny how he handles it. He says: "The process is the same. All these drugs perturb neurotransmitter systems and the brain compensates. The difference is, with illicit drugs, that ends up with addiction. With licit drugs, that ends up with a therapeutic outcome." So, anyway ....

I also heard another description of how you can distinguish between licit and illicit drugs. Illicit drugs people will pay for themselves. Legal drugs will only be taken if someone else is paying for them.

## Mainstream Biological Psychiatry

Now, imagine I'm a mainstream biological psychiatrist and I'm giving this talk and I'm going to present the evidence for both short-term and long-term use. What is the mainstream psychiatric establishment saying about its evidence base? Because if you were to go to an American Psychiatric Association conference, they would say, "Our evidence base is great; it's solid. We are following the evidence."

First, they have short-term trials. Let's say you take people with psychotic symptoms as they enter the emergency room or whatever. You do studies where you take one group that is put on antipsychotics, the other group on placebo. And what the researchers would report is that the group treated with medication, at least on their scales, had a decrease in psychotic symptoms better than the placebo group over six weeks. Okay? So that ostensibly showed short-term efficacy.

# Anatomy of an Epidemic

Now, in *Anatomy of an Epidemic*, I'm not questioning any of these studies. What David Healy did with the antidepressants yesterday was to say, you really have to question the short term efficacy of the antidepressants, and I don't do this in the book. I'm just saying, here's what they did. In short term studies, they invented their scales and on those scales the drug shows some benefit over placebo in knocking down the target symptom of the disease. Now, historically once you get people on a medication, you have to figure out how long they should be on it. Right? And a lot of the keeping-people-on-medication-for-life paradigm arose from the antipsychotic studies. They did trials like this. They would take those patients who stabilized well on the meds. And you have to take people who stabilized well, as they have to be fairly nonpsychotic when they enter the relapse studies. So researchers would take the 40% or so who a year after initial treatment are still doing pretty well and then they would run trials that were designed like this: half of the patients would be abruptly withdrawn and half would be maintained on the drug.

With the group that was withdrawn, it was abrupt withdrawal, and consequently they relapsed at a much higher rate. So that was seen, particularly in the 1960s and 1970s, as evidence that staying on the drug prevented the return of the disease. Do you see that? That's really the evidence base for psychotropic drugs. It's short-term trials and relapse trials. And sure enough, once people are on and you take people off the medication, particularly if you do it abruptly as most of these studies did, the group coming off relapses at a higher rate. (Viguera, 1998).

As I followed this, I now understood those two parts of their evidence base. But what is missing from these data is the long-term evidence base. Can you see what's missing? Does that tell you anything about employment? Does it tell you anything about functioning? And you can see the flaw also in their relapse studies. Is that high relapse rate really the return of the disease or is it due to the fact that the brain has been changed and now you're withdrawing the drug? Right? And, in fact, in 1995, Patricia Gilbert summarized the relapse studies for the antipsychotics, and she said, you know, the relapse rate is like three times higher for those medications withdrawn and this is the solid evidence we have for keeping schizophrenia patients on the drugs forever. Then a gentleman named Ross Baldessarini (1995), a researcher from Harvard Medical School, said: Wait a minute. These are mostly abrupt trials. Can we find some gradual trials? There have been very few gradual withdrawal trials. He sort of identified a few, and in those, the relapse rate was only about half as much as in the abrupt withdrawal trials. So you clearly saw that part of that high relapse rate was in fact drug-related (Viguera, 1997).

The next thing I looked at was that this doesn't tell us the long-term course. Imagine that we have 100 patients come in to the emergency room. We put 50 on the drug and we put 50 on the nondrug or other treatment and then we follow them for two, three years. This evidence base doesn't tell how those two groups would be different two or three years later. Right? So one of the things I looked at as I was doing this book was whether mainstream psychiatry has evidence that it is really shifting the long-term outcomes of major mental disorders for the better. What I found is confusing, as we don't have that evidence.

So, for example, Stip (2002) basically reviewed this question regarding antipsychotics. He asked whether fifty years after the introduction of antipsychotics if we have evidence that these drugs are effective? His conclusion was that over the long term, there is no compelling evidence. Then he went on to say that if we want psychiatry to be evidence-based and we take a closer look at this evidence base, we need to be ready to be surprised. Now, why was this important for me to find? It was like the green light that there is something to be found out there. We can try to put together this picture of how drugs affect long-term outcomes. That meant I wouldn't be missing something. Right? Because Stip had looked and he hadn't found the evidence for how drugs shift outcomes long term.

How do you put together a picture? How did I try to put together a picture? I do it for four major mental disorders, and what we're going to do real quickly is go through it for depression, since this was a psychotherapy conference where a lot of focus is obviously on depression. We'll do it for depression, a little bit for bipolar. But in the book, I do it for schizophrenia, anxiety, bipolar, and depression, and then I also do it for kids, try to look at what's happening with kids. But how do you put together the picture? Here's what I did, since I think this is important from a logical point of view.

First, I wanted to see what the epidemiological studies were telling us about this disorder before the revolution occurred. So what was the prevalence of these disorders and what was the long-term outcome? This makes sense, as you're going to see a baseline.

## What Did Physicians See at the Beginning?

The next thing I wanted to look at was whether physicians who were around when the drugs were introduced, did they see something different in the clinical course of their patients? Because, remember, they have the experience where they've seen what happens to major depressed patients who weren't put on medication, whereas the doctors today don't have that. The ability to see that is lost. I wanted to see, when the drugs are introduced, what doctors were saying about the long-term course. Then if there were any randomized studies that lasted longer, a year or two or three, I would try to find those.

The next thing I wanted to find is, as they do modern epidemiological studies, what is the long-term course, and how does that compare back in the pre era when the disorders were running a more chronic course than today. I'm going to use the epidemiological surveys to compare. Then I'm going to look to see if there is a moment in the literature in which mainstream guys ask, "What in the hell was going on?" I want to see if they saw that, and if they did, was it a biological explanation they came up with for what was going on.

And then finally I was going to try to find what are called "naturalistic longitudinal studies," in which you just follow people, starting from initial cohorts in that some people will just go off meds, and then just look who does better at five years, ten years, etc.

Now, when you do that, here's what I think you find. Over the long term, in the paradigm of care in the aggregate you see a worsening of the target symptoms; and I'll show you some of these data. In other words, depressed patients who are long term on meds are more likely to still be depressed five years later, ten years later than the unmedicated group. It actually is the same with the psychotic patients. You actually see a lot more psychosis longitudinally with long-term use of the medication. And I'll show you a study that really brings that home.

With bipolar episodes, you actually see a lot more rapid cycling, a lot more mood instability today than you used to see fifty years ago. So I think one thing you'll see in the data is actually worsening of the target symptoms. That does not mean that nobody does well on the drugs. I think that some people, as John, said 9 to 15% are good responders to the drug. I think you have to acknowledge that, as there are some good responders. But what we're talking about here is how are outcomes shaped in the aggregate? For example, if you have a disorder where 70% get better naturally or, without drugs, and now only 50% get better on the drugs, you're still lowering the overall outcome. Okay? Does that make sense? That's the first thing I think you'll see.

The second thing I do think you'll see is that in a certain percentage of people, you get new and more severe symptoms. You get some physical problems, you get some emotional problems, and at least for some of the drugs you'll see some cognitive problems. You'll see that with the long term.

And then finally you see basically what shows up over and over again, that there is the risk of early death that increases with the long-term use of antidepressants.

Anyway, that's the summary, and are there data that support those conclusions?

## Depression before and after Antidepressants.

Depression in the pre-antidepressant era, who did it affect in prevalence? Basically, if you look at 1955, 90% of the first admissions to public and private hospitals for depression were 35 years and older. In other words, depression in 1955 was basically a middle-age disorder. People under 30 got anxious, not depressed. In terms of the prevalence, it was roughly one in one thousand adults that had a bout of major depression each year, making it a fairly rare disorder.

Short-term outcomes in the pre-antidepressant era in hospitalized populations were that the depression could be expected to lift. But if you look in terms of three months, four months, five months, six months, eight months, most people were getting out of the hospital within those time periods. At the start of the antidepressant era, here is what people were saying. Jonathan Cole (1964) from the NIMH, stated, "Depression is, on the whole, one of the psychiatric conditions with the best prognosis for eventual recovery with or without treatment. Most depressions are self-limiting." In other words, if you get a bout you will soon recover from it. Nathan Kline (1964), in the *Journal of the American Medical Association* said, "In the treatment of depression, one always has an ally in the fact that most depressions terminate in spontaneous remissions." This means that in many cases regardless of what one does the patient will eventually get better." Because of this understanding of depression, do you know why antidepressants were first introduced? It was to hasten recovery. Yes, the idea was to speed up recovery.

What were the long-term outcomes of depression? As Silverman (1968) reported, a study in Germany found that 60% of 450 of patients hospitalized for a bout of depression had only that one bout. Only 13% had to be rehospitalized two or three times in their entire lives. There were other studies like that of Horatio Pollock in 1931 in New York State, another one in Sweden (Gunnar Lundquist, 1945), and if you put all these together you really find out about the course of major depression prior to the antidepressant era. It's like this: with people serious enough to be hospitalized for major depression, 50% would get out of the hospital and never be re-hospitalized in these long-term studies. About another 30% you see that they might have a second episode or a third episode. And it was really only about 20% that were becoming chronically ill. So it was seen mostly as an episodic illness, and not as a chronic illness.

Now, what happened once the drugs were introduced? What did clinicians notice? Right away you started hearing this from physicians: My patients are getting better faster, but it seems like they're now relapsing more frequently. In other words, the recurrence of depression is increasing. Instead of people staying well two years, three years, or extended periods, it seems as if when they go on the drug, they get a little better, but when they off the drug, they would relapse right away. A researcher in the Netherlands (Van Scheyen, 1973) tested this out. For two years, he studied 94 depressed patients and concluded that more systematic long-term antidepressant medication, with or without ECT, exerts a paradoxical effect on the recurrent nature of their vital depression. In other words, this therapeutic approach was associated with an increase in recurrent rate and a decrease in cycle duration. This was especially true in female patients. Should this increase be regarded as an untoward long-term side effect of treatment with tricyclic antidepressants?

The point here is that right from the beginning of the psychotropic era you hear this uh-oh moment, that maybe we're increasing the chronicity of this disorder.

At this point there are a lot of relapse studies being done, and eventually they found out, as did Ross Baldessarini (2007) of Harvard Medical School, that 50% of all depressed patients that are put on an antidepressant and withdrawn from it relapse within 14 months. So this constitutes a much greater relapse for as you will remember, it used to be 50% would stay well indefinitely and 20–30% that would probably stay well two, three years, etc. So now, after exposure, 50% are having a relapse within 14 months. But there is another thing that's happening. That 50% was in people medicated and then coming off. The relapse rate was lower for those stayed on the drug in some of these trials. But, nevertheless, they began to notice when they followed people long term that they were relapsing with greater frequency. It seems like with the drug, the disorder was turning chronic. Finally the editor of the journal *Psychotherapy and Psychosomatics*, Giovanni Fava (1994), raised this key question: Are these drugs depressogenic over the long term? The reason this question is so profound, when you have drugs, you need a risk-benefit analysis in regard to the target symptoms. In other words, we've got to knock down the target symptom better than placebo as that will justify all the risks and all the adversities. If we're getting greater depression over the long term, we're losing the benefit side of that—that equation. So justifiably, he raises this issue of whether the drugs are depressogenic? Again, Ross Baldessarini as sort of the father of American psychopharmacology, said this is an important question. It's not one we want to have to face, but it's one that we should face. What happens in response? Donald Kline, who I think was at Columbia University, says to Giovanni Fava in a public forum, stop asking this question. Nobody is interested. The NIMH is not interested, the pharmaceutical companies are not interested, and basically the APA is not interested. Do you see the betrayal in that? What does everyone want to know when they start the antidepressant? Yeah, they want to get out of the depression, but they also want to know what might be happening to them long term. Basically this is saying "we're not going to investigate that." Anyway, my point here is, this arose within the literature, this sort of fear of what's happening. Then I looked at the epidemiological studies and saw that these studies were showing that depression was running a much more chronic course. As early as 1985, the NIMH convened a little panel on this, and they noticed this problem: All early epidemiological studies showed depression ran at a pretty benign long-term course, while modern ones were showing a much more chronic course. What did they do? Well, what they said was that those old studies must have been flawed. That's how they explained it away. They said that an improvement in science tells us now what the real course of depression is. But what are they really seeing? They're seeing the course of medicated depression. They also said we now believe that most patients would eventually recover from a major depressive episode because that's what they saw in their hospitalized cohorts. They did recover and they got out and many of them did not come back. Now they say that more extensive studies prove the assumption that depression is a highly recurrent and pernicious disorder. That's the shift from the pre-medicated era to the medicated era.

So, I hope you see what I'm doing in this. I'm following their studies and their sort of insights. Now, you can either buy that it was all about the epidemiological studies being just flawed, or not. But at least it is apparent there is a recognition that the epidemiological studies have changed.

## The Fallacy of the Star*D Trial.

Now, you might have heard of the Star*D Trial. How many of you have ever heard of the Star*D Trial? This was a really key trial, biggest, largest antidepressant trial ever run: 4041 patients. It was done by the NIMH. And if you listen to the press releases and if you go talk to your average doctor, they will tell you that study worked. What they will tell you is that 67% of the patients who entered that study remitted. And here is how the study was done. You were put on a first antidepressant. And if you didn't remit on that, you went to a second antidepressant. If you didn't remit on that, you went to a third antidepressant. If you didn't remit on that, you went to a fourth antidepressant. And what they said was that by the end of the fourth stage, 67% of people were remitted. Symptoms were gone. And thus it became evidence for the treatment of depression. If the first antidepressant doesn't work, keep trying the second one, third one, and a fourth one and you will eventually find one that works. I was at my tennis club the other day listening to a couple of doctors talk, "Ah, yeah, we know our antidepressants work because of the Star*D Trial."

This trial is one of the most corrupt, it is so bad (source, Pigott, 2010). First of all, it was the way they got to that 67%. If people had stayed in the trial from Stage 1 to Stage 2 and remitted at the same rate as those who did stay in the trial, we would have got this 67% remission rate. That's number one.

Number two is, they changed outcome measures. They moved from the Hamilton scale to these other measures.

Number three is, they were enrolling people and counting them as patients who by their own study criteria weren't depressed enough to be enrolled in this trial in the first place. So they were including in this remission rate people who had a score of fewer than 14 on the Hamilton scale that has an entry requirement of 14 or above to be considered depressed. But they had to have a certain number of patients, so they enrolled these unqualified people anyway and included them.

There has been some reanalysis of these data. In fact, David did some of this reanalysis. What are the real data? Well, first of all, only 38% of the patients properly enrolled in the trial remitted during one of the four stages of drug treatment. That's when you see those who actually remitted. So 38% who had a score of above 14 on it remitted during one of those four stages. The rest either dropped out or didn't remit. But it's the second number that is the key. Only 3% of the 4000 patients who entered this trial remitted and stayed well and in the trial for as long as a year. And they were being paid like 25 bucks or whatever to stay in the trial. As far as I know, that's the worst stay-well rate I've ever seen in any trial anywhere of antidepressants.

So this sort of goes to what David Healy was saying yesterday. This was NIMH's big trial to figure out how effective antidepressants really are. The message that went out to the public was that 67% remitted, and their symptoms vanished. What really happened? Only 3% stabilized, which is a bit of a difference. Now, the rest either didn't remit or dropped out, that sort of thing.

## What Naturalistic Studies Tend to Show

Okay, the last thing I did here was try to look at naturalistic studies. I looked at every naturalistic study I could find. The first one was a 10-year study of depression in the Netherlands (Weel-Baumgarten, 2000). You'll see that those who were treated without a drug, close to 80% never had another episode in the course of ten years, whereas those treated with a drug, only

50% stayed well during the ten years. By the way, that's actually a pretty good stay-well rate for those treated with antidepressants. It's just not nearly as good as those being treated without the antidepressant. See the difference? But that stay-well rate is pretty common to those in the old pre-medicated era.

Next was a one-year outcome in a World Health Organization (WHO) screening study for depression (Goldberg, 1998). This was done in fifteen cities around the world. Here was their hypothesis, that those diagnosed and treated would have better outcomes. People are coming into clinics for all sorts of problems, and the WHO researchers would identify people with depression, but they would not diagnose them. They would wait and see if the regular doctor diagnosed them as depressed. The theory was that those diagnosed and treated would have the better one-year outcomes. And this study in fifteen cities was going to prove the value of screening for depression. That was the hypothesis. What were the outcomes? Those most likely to still be depressed at the end of one year were those diagnosed and treated with antidepressants. So they were most likely to still be depressed at the end of one year. Less likely were diagnosed and treated with benzos (benzodiazepine). The third was those who were undiagnosed and were given no drugs. The least likely were those who were diagnosed, but were given no drugs. In other words, it was the non-medicated patients that had the lowest level of continuing depression at the end of one year. So, it then noted this did not support the value of screening for depression and then treating with drugs.

A really interesting study was done by in Ontario by Carolyn Dewa (2003). In Canada, if you've missed work for ten days due to depression you go on to short-term disability. Now the question is: In the next six months are you going to return to work or you go on to long-term disability? What they found was that in some ways, this shows that the drugs work. 71% of those who took an antidepressant returned to work and did not go on to long-term disability. Now, I'm willing to bet that if you ask those people, they would say that medications work. They would be voices for saying how helpful antidepressants are. And maybe they were, as those people did go back to work. Maybe this does show a real use. Nevertheless, those who didn't take the medication had an even higher return to work rate. And if you look at the disability numbers, 19% of those who were treated with an antidepressant went on to long-term disability versus 9% of those who did not.

Now, the caveat with naturalistic studies is that maybe those who are not medicated aren't as ill in the beginning. And maybe they have a different inner resilience, so you have that caveat as well. But, nevertheless, you see some consistency with these data of an increased risk of disability.

Now, this is an important study. This is a six-year study. Beginning in 1978, the NIMH launched a very big study called The Psychobiology of Depression Research Study, for which there have been a number of spinoff studies. One of these spin-offs was in the 1990s (Coryell, 1995) and it raised the question of what is the course of un-medicated depression today? This six-year study found that 32% of the treated group had a cessation of role functioning, which basically meant either they quit being able to work as a housewife or in a job, whereas only 10% of those who weren't treated became incapacitated. Disability was seven times higher for the treated group. So, again, in all these naturalistic studies, you see lower disability rates for the untreated group.

Finally, there was this study done by Duke University with the hypothesis that exercise plus a drug would have a cumulative benefit (Babyak, 2000). At the end of 16 weeks, in fact, the drug patients did do a little bit better than the exercise-only patients. But at the end of 10 months the exercise only group was doing the best. In other words, 30% of the exercise-alone group was still depressed at the end of 10 months, whereas roughly over half of those with drug or drug plus exercise were depressed. It seems that the drug is an anchor that is weighing down the recovery rate of those with exercise. That is exactly the opposite of what they hypothesized.

## Bipolar Disorder

The bipolar story is somewhat similar. If you look at long-term outcomes with bipolar, where did all the bipolar patients come from? Bipolar was a rare disorder in the pre-drug era (Lundquist, 1945; Tsuang, 1979) as David Healy knows quite well as you came up with one in five thousand people as the prevalence. So assume one in five thousand people had bipolar illness that in 1950–1955 was called manic-depression. Today, it's one in fifty in the United States. There was some data the other day that maybe it's one in twenty-five. So how did it go from one in five thousand to one in fifty? This is what was really stirring this disability upswing. And the answer is that there are really four gateways to that. One is the old way. There are some people that show these up-and-down cycles, and that's a small percentage. You might call that organic bipolar or something. And then it is illicit drugs, such as marijuana. So you will see an increased risk with regular use of marijuana, especially, I think, the marijuana of today which is more potent. If you survey all bipolar patients, about 25% today would say they had used marijuana. So about 25% of patients will tell you they had their first psychotic episode while doing marijuana. And there was a recent study that says, yes, that increases the risk.

The second is antidepressants. So it's real clear that the risk of moving from unipolar to bipolar is increased once you're on an antidepressant. The best study I saw of this was by Yale University investigators. They looked into a database of roughly ninety thousand people and they looked at those who were treated with an antidepressant and those who were not, and they said the conversion rate is about three times higher. So you see the risk there.

And then finally there has been an expansion of the diagnostics. It used to be, to get a manic-depressive illness, you had to be hospitalized for both poles (i.e., mania and depression). Now you don't have to be hospitalized and to get bipolar II you don't have to be hospitalized for either pole. They have shortened the time you have to be manic or depressed. And as you know, it is sort of the diagnosis of the day; you can get diagnosed if you're just a little bit too moody sometimes. But that's a diagnosis that comes with a sense of lifelong medication. So by expanding that diagnostics, you were inviting people into a serious category with a serious use of drugs.

In terms of bipolar outcomes, basically you used to see what was described as an episodic illness. People would say they would have the manic episode or the depressive episode, and it would pass. They would recover to what is known as euthymia, an absence of symptoms. And roughly it would go like this, and there would be no functional decline during that time. Furthermore, basically 50% of the cohort hospitalized would never be re-hospitalized. About 30% would have these periodic episodes, like a flu that would revisit every two, three, four years, and only about 20% would be chronically ill. The functional outcome was that 70% to 80% would be working long term, with no long-term cognitive decline. What do you find today? As soon as antidepressants are introduced, you start seeing that people are saying these episodes are becoming more frequent and you see people complaining about rapid cycles. So it's the same sort of thing we have already looked at.

Look at what they were saying about manic-depressive illness in the pre-drug era: There is no basis to consider that manic-depressive psychosis permanently affected those who suffered from it. In this way, it is of course different from schizophrenia. While some people suffered multiple episodes, each episode was usually only "a few months in duration" and in a significant number of patients, only one episode of illness occurs. Once patients recover, they usually had "no difficulty resuming their usual occupations."

Fred Goodwin (2005), former director of NIMH, stated what may be regarded as a summary: "If you create a patient in this way with use of antidepressants, even when you remove the antidepressants, you may still have this person who has been destabilized." So you see the risk.

The drugs are introduced and what are people saying? The general impression today is that the course of recurrence is happening more. So you see the same thing, the sense that we're getting more episodes. This is the course of the day. In epidemiological studies, you see more recurrent episodes, more rapid cycling. Instead of recovering in between episodes, if you look at diaries of bipolar patients, you'll see a lot of low-level depression. We're getting some long-term cognitive impairment and we're getting some physical problems.

Here's what I think is key. Just read these three statements. These are not by critics. Carlos Zarate (2000) headed the NIMH mood disorders program. What did he say? Outcome used to be good and not so good today. Ross Baldessarini (1995) is like the father of American psychopharmacology. What is he saying? Outcomes used to be good and they're not so good today. I mean, his is a little bit ironic. Prognosis for bipolar disorder was once considered relatively favorable, but contemporary findings suggest that disability and poor outcomes are prevalent despite major therapeutic advances. I'm not sure why the course would run— worse course if you have major therapeutic advances.

My point is this, even though I rushed through the bipolar data, there is a recognition of the deterioration of this by the mainstream guys. And the real tragedy we have here is that functional outcomes for bipolar patients in terms of long-term employment are down to about 33% in the United States, from 80%. Do you know what the real tragedy is also? They didn't used to show cognitive impairment. They are now starting to show cognitive impairment after about five years on meds. And long-term bipolar outcomes are beginning to merge with schizophrenia. That's how bad bipolar outcomes have deteriorated. And if you want to know why this is so, just look at the use of atypical antipsychotics in the population. There was a recent study that showed basically that these medications shrink the brain over time. And if you follow that through, that shrinkage is associated with increased functional impairment, greater lethargy, and in fact cognitive impairment. So, it's what you expect if you're using antipsychotics on bipolar patients.

## Antipsychotics and Schizophrenia.

If anything needs to be addressed, it's this. Where do all the bipolar patients come from and why are the outcomes so poor? And of course, then, we can look at kids and wonder about that as well. Okay. I know I'm hitting you with a lot of stuff here today. I'm just going to do this one last thing with schizophrenia. If there should be anything that we are supposed to be absolutely sure of is that antipsychotics improve the long-term course of schizophrenia. Our society is set up to insist that people stay on antipsychotics, but there's a whole long story that tells you something quite different. If you really go back and look at schizophrenia outcomes and psychotic episodes in the pre-drug era, you find there were many people that "descended into schizophrenia and got better" after a year or two years. In fact, if you go back to 1945–1955, the employment rates for first-episode schizophrenia patients five years out were above 50%. So this idea that nobody can work or be employed is not really shown in those data. This is the last study and then I'll conclude my presentation.

Martin Harrow (2007) is psychologist at the University of Illinois, College of Medicine who did a study that is unique in our literature. It is a very interesting study. From 1978–1981, he went to two hospitals and he enrolled about two hundred psychotic patients into his study. He followed one-hundred forty-five for fifteen years, which is a low drop-out rate for a fifteen year study. He ended up with sixty-four schizophrenic patients, and eighty-one people with milder disorders whom he had followed for fifteen years. And what he did was just a naturalistic study. Everybody was treated with drugs in the hospital. There's no randomization. He just followed up how they were doing at two, four-and-a-half, seven, ten, and fifteen years. He looked at whether they're still in the hospital, are they working, are they asymptomatic, and are they using drugs? The expectation of course is that the medicated patients will do much better. This is a young group, by the way, mostly with their first episode, and with an average age of twenty-two. I honestly believe this is the only study to be found in which a cohort of patients with medication use that were tracked this long. This would be true for bipolar patients, or for anybody, as I don't know of another study like this. What do you see here? The so-called unmedicated group that was twenty-five of the sixty-four schizophrenic patients was off antipsychotics at the end of two years. Twenty of the sixty-four are off all meds, while there were five taking some meds. Anyway, they're doing slightly better at the end of two years in terms of the recovery rate. But between two and four-and-a-half years, the off-med group does much better. It continues to get better, such that, by the end of four-and-a-half-years 40% of those off meds are in recovery versus only 5% of those on meds. And that difference in recovery rate stayed that way throughout the fifteen years of follow up.

The next bit of data looked at all patients in regard to global adjustment. As we saw, at the end of two years the off-med group is just doing a little bit better than the on-med group. But what happens between two years and four-and-a-half years? The off-med group continues to get better, where the on-med group does not. That is a very statistically significant difference between those two in terms of global functioning. Other studies don't capture this time frame. Those six-week studies and those withdrawal studies do not capture this.

Harrow's study had basically three outcome categories: recovered, so-so, and uniformly poor. Here's how the results went. Of the off-medicated group, 40% were in the recovered category; 44% were in the so-so; 16% in were uniformly poor. The on-med group was 5% recovered, 45% roughly so-so, and 49% uniformly poor. So what do you see there? It's almost as if you see a shift to chronicity, right? Almost half the medicated group had the worst outcomes, which only belies everything that we all are supposed to know about antipsychotics. Which group was most likely to still be suffering from antipsychotic symptoms? It was those who were still taking the drug. Remember what I told you about how medications seem to shape long-term outcomes and even on the target symptom? Look at which group is more actively psychotic after ten and fifteen years. There were many more actively psychotic in the on medication group.

Now, remember, Harrow has a second group of patients, those with milder psychotic disorders. How they did on global adjustment are the data I would like to show American psychiatry. They need to look at this at grand rounds. In fact, I presented this at MGH Grand Rounds. What do we see there? You see the best group is the milder disorders who are off meds. What is the second best group? It is schizophrenics who are off meds. Now, how does schizophrenia off meds end up better than milder disorders on meds? Which group had the better prognosis since day one, milder disorders or schizophrenia? Milder, of course. Well, why did the schizophrenia off meds end up better? And I would say all of you going into this field should try to grapple with why that might be.

In Martin Harrow's story, what is the response from mainstream psychiatry? If you read his article, he explains the results by stating these were just good prognosis patients who were able to get off meds. The drugs work, he and his collaborators said. Everyone stabilized. They help people stabilize and there were these good prognosis patients who then got off and did well. So it's just a matter that there is self-selection going on and there is this subset that can do well off meds. That's the discussion in the published article. So I said to Martin Harrow, "That's not what your data show. Your milder patients off drugs do better than your milder patients on. The schizophrenia off drugs as a whole did better than your schizophrenia on." Then I said, "Your good prognosis patients off drugs did better than your good prognosis patients on. How do you explain that, that crossing of schizophrenia off and milder disorders on?" He got furious with me, to be honest with you. Here's what he said. "I was told not to publish this. This was bad for psychopharm." And then he said, basically, he thought his funding would be threatened by publishing this. What he was telling me was that he had to put a spin on this in his written article so as to avoid highlighting these data. These data are from his data tables, as he doesn't write in his article that the schizophrenia patients off meds did better than his milder disorders on meds. He does not say that. Rather, it is spun in a different way. Why is this? These results seem impossible. It just seems like it can't be.

Well, I would tell you that there two other things in the biological literature that might explain this. One is the increase in the D2 receptors. Well, there's a guy who's doing animal research, Philip Seeman at the University of Toronto. He's doing animal models of psychosis. He gives them amphetamines, he gives them angel dust, he does some gene knockout studies, and he says, for whatever reason, all of these pathways to psychosis converge with one final thing. They all cause an increase in D2 receptors that have a high affinity for dopamine. That's the common biological marker. Now guess what. If you give olanzapine or Haldol to a person, it causes the same thing. It doubles the number of high-density D2 receptors. So what Seeman says is: That's why the drugs lose their effectiveness. What he's not saying is that you're basically causing the same biological problem you see in animal models with psychoses. Yet there is a line of thinking in the literature, going back to the 1980s that the drugs make you extra vulnerable to psychosis over time. That may be what we're seeing.

The other thing you may be seeing is suggested in a study by Nancy Andreasen (2005) that I would urge all of you to read. You can get this on my website at www.madinamerica.com. Who is Nancy Andreasen? She wrote *The Broken Brain*. Okay? So she helped set up this medical model. She was editor of the *American Journal of Psychiatry* from 1993 to 2005. In the early 1990s, she began an MRI study, a big study of about five hundred first-episode schizophrenia patients. And her theory, her model was that schizophrenia is a neurodegenerative disease characterized by brain volume loss over time. So she did the MRIs and she found that in fact there is this tissue loss, like 1% a year, and it's somewhat notable in the frontal lobes. And then she did a study that showed that as this tissue loss happens, we get increased functional impairments, we get increased negative symptoms, and we get cognitive decline. So her model now is this. This is the disease and the drugs fail to stop that process. She had an interview with the *New York Times* in 2008 in which she said: "But we do know that the more drugs you're given, the more tissue you lose," and that's a model that shows the drugs exacerbate that process. If you give antipsychotics to macaque monkeys, their brains will shrink. And finally, I think it was about a month ago that she published a paper that said: The shrinkage does not correlate with illness or severity. It does not correlate with substance abuse. It correlates with drug, amounts of drug. The more drug you're given, the more the shrinkage. So you see the problem with this? That is a story of the long term usage. The medication does seem to work over the short term. It helps people stabilize. Right? And some people may do well long term on antipsychotics, so you can find a use for them. But long term it's telling you, at the very least there's this worry that the drugs cause a morphological change that makes you more vulnerable to psychosis and causes these other impairments.

Finally, so as to conclude my presentation on a moment of optimism, I refer to Western Lapland, a part of Finland that, beginning in 1992, rethought their use of antipsychotics. And what they do is this. They believe in family therapy as well as a form of psychotherapy that is called open dialogue therapy there. There is a long history behind this. It began in 1969, and here's what they do. When people come to them with a first psychotic episode, they do not put them on antipsychotics. They want to see if they can get people well without causing that brain change. Doesn't that make sense? They throw a lot of resources into treating these first-episode people. However, if someone isn't getting better within the first three or four weeks, then they use the drugs.

Long-term outcomes are this, as reported by Seikkula (2006). At the end of five years, 80% of their patients are either working or back in school. Only 20% have gone on to long-term disability. Their unemployment rate for that 80% is lower than it is for the Finnish population as a whole. That shows they are really working at getting people back to work. And in terms of drug use, 33% of their patients have been exposed to antipsychotics in that five years, meaning 2/3 have never been exposed and only 20% are regularly maintained on them. Now, what I love about this story is that it's not an anti-medication story. It is a best-use story. If I gave you a talk just about antipsychotics, you would see a lot of research that supports this model of care, which says you want to see if you can get people through the psychotic episode without putting them on drugs. If there's a chance that people can get better and not go down this very long-term problematic course that is desirable. But at the same time, it's saying that the drugs have some use for a certain population.

This pertains to what John talked about, and this goes to the entire subject of antidepressants, mood stabilizers, the whole gamut, asking for whom and for how long? Those are the questions that have to be raised. And I think what all these data don't say is that there's no place for medications in psychiatry. There's clearly a place for short-term use, and some people appear to do well on them long term. But the paradigm of care that we have that says use them right away and keep people on them long term, that's, as I see it, is not what these data are telling us. We are applying a broken paradigm of care and we're now applying this broken paradigm of care to kids. You really have to ask, if you see all this chronicity, you see all this cognitive decline, good God, what are we doing to the kids, especially with the use of antipsychotics? Anyway, thank you.

MODERATOR (Dr. O'Donohue): Okay. We now have time for a couple of questions or comments. If you'd like to raise your hand, we'll get a microphone to you.

QUESTIONER ONE: Thanks for the talk. It was great. Your book is great too. But I'm wondering how much of problems with long-term outcome you think are really due to changes from the medication use versus just a change in how the person perceives him or herself?

MR. WHITAKER: That's a great question.

QUESTIONER ONE: You know, once they're labeled with the diagnosis and medication treatment plan and so forth?

MR. WHITAKER: Do you all understand this question? This is a great question. It's a really profound question, actually.

What happens in the course following the diagnosis? As you know, I interviewed perhaps ninety people who were diagnosed while I was writing this book, especially many people who were diagnosed when they were eighteen to twenty. You know what I heard over and over again? "I got diagnosed and then I had to deal with the crushing hopelessness that my life was over." This is sort of what you're getting at here: that I have a broken brain, I'm not a full person, and I have to deal with these drugs. And that can become a self-fulfilling prophecy. It also is a very disempowering message because you're telling them that you can't do anything. In other words, you can just take your drugs and supposedly that's going to fix things. But that's not really encouraging one to make life changes, to exercise, to go out and make friends.

I think the antipsychotics clearly have some iatrogenic long-term effects. There are also some iatrogenic short-term effects, the metabolic problems, and that sort of thing. So, I think the fact that the brain is shrinking is not good in general. But I think that may be a big part of the antidepressants, to be honest with you. I mean, I don't really know, but certainly it's sort of a depressing thing to be told you have a chronic illness.

With the mood stabilizers for bipolar, you know, again, you're told you have a chronic illness and that this is a serious illness. That's pretty pessimistic. I know a lot of people on single antidepressants, or monotherapy, for bipolar that seem to be doing quite well. But people on cocktails really seem to wind up with a problematic course, where they're shifting all the time. They stay well for a little while only.

Anyway, I don't know the answer to the question, but I think it's part of it and actually it is part of the problem. Personally, I think you need to totally shift the paradigm of care this way. You need to have psychosocial care as the centerpiece, addressing how do we all stay healthy? We need friendships, we need meaning in our life, we need someone to love, and we need someone to love us. You make that the centerpiece of what you try to restore and keep, and then you figure out how the drugs over here as a tool can be best used. If you have that paradigm of care, you're not delivering this pessimistic message because you're not saying they have broken brain, you're not saying necessarily you have to use the medications for life. You have over here this tool that maybe when you figure out how to use it for whom and for how long. That's your good sensible question. I think that's a big problem with this paradigm of care. It's so pessimistic.

QUESTIONER TWO: Who's been most receptive and who has been most opposed to your book?

MR. WHITAKER: As you might imagine, this has been something of a controversial book and there's been some pretty slashing attacks. I mean, I woke up the day the book was published to open the *Boston Globe* and there was a review in which I was compared to an AIDS denier and a South African dictator who had caused the death of hundreds of thousands of people. This is not a great way to wake up.

That was a bad start for my book. But actually things began to shift, and I'm increasingly being asked to speak to professional audiences. I think the most hopeful thing that's happened, people began calling me up, saying, "Wow, we really haven't looked at long-term outcomes. We really need to think about this and put things together." This includes psychiatrists, administrators, and some psychologists. They had a meeting in Oregon in early February that was led by a psychiatrist. There were four workshops: one on schizophrenia, one on depression, one on medication tapering, and one that included someone from the federal government on how to basically get Medicaid waivers and Medicaid payments for this sort of thing. There were fifty people from seventeen states, and they came up with a consensus statement. These psychiatrists said the data show that with a first episode, we shouldn't be putting everybody on antipsychotics. Now, I don't know if that sounds radical or not, but that's actually radical in terms of practices. And they said the reason is because the long-term data show that there's a subset that can get better without antipsychotics and you want to make that possible.

The schizophrenia consensus statement was led by two psychiatrists with Harvard Medical School affiliations. There were also a couple academic doctors from the Oregon Health Sciences University, who had also looked at the long-term data. They had looked at the Harrow data. They had looked at the Soteria data. There's a long history of literature that tells a story. They also said that every schizophrenia patient should have a chance to go off meds, because you have to allow for this possibility. And that would mean supporting their going off in safe environments. That's a pretty radical thing if you could actually implement that in the protocols. And there's a foundation that has now formed that's raising money. It's called The Foundation for Excellence in Mental Healthcare. I helped form it and then I retreated from it. I didn't want to be part of it for journalistic reasons. It's raising money. It has some psychiatrists on the board. It has the former state commissioner of Oregon Mental Health on the board. It has the current Director of Association of Community Mental Health Programs in Oregon on the board. It's really trying to be a mainstream group, and they are trying to do two things. One of the problems that we have talked about is information. We have 80% of Americans thinking that chemical imbalances cause mental disorders. How many of you know the Harrow Study? How many of you know those data? How many of you knew those data before today? Why didn't you? I'm serious. Why didn't you know those data? Did you know that the recovery rate of the best long-term study we have was 5% for those off meds and 40% for those on meds? Why wasn't that publicized?

Well, when Harrow published this study, did the APA put out a press release? No. Did the NIMH put out a press release? No. Did NAMI put out a press release? No. Do you know what psychiatric residents now learn about this study? There's a line in the book that says: The Harrow study shows there's a small group of people with schizophrenia who can do okay without the continued benefit of antipsychotics. That's not what that study shows. It raises a lot more questions than that. So, anyway, this foundation wants to become an information source, an honest information source.

In addition, they want to fund research so if people want to do a pilot project such as one where they would go to Finland, figure out what they're doing there and then replicate it here. They want to put up a fund to do that and then chart those outcomes. So they want to actually build a new evidence base, which in essence is what they're talking about. It would be an evidence base that incorporates long-term data. And I will tell you; the beauty of this story is that there is an optimistic story to be discovered in the long-term outcome statements. And the optimistic story is that we have this crazy thing right now we call mental illness and what we call normal, and you can cross over that line from mental illness back to normal. Do you know what I mean? Also, if you have the right stresses, you can move over here, from the normal side of the line, to the psychiatric distress side of the line. But even with psychosis, with the right psychosocial support and probably the right judicious use of medication, people can get back to the normal side. And they're not chronically ill, they're not mentally ill for the rest of their lives. They may have had a manic episode or depressive episode or even a psychotic episode. But many people can leave it behind. And that's sort of the optimism to be discovered and that's what this foundation wants to do. It wants to show that here's the long-term outcomes literature, and it wants to sponsor pilot projects that will augment and support that.

That foundation also had a depression workshop. Do you know what they concluded after looking at the long-term outcomes literature? Well, (a) you shouldn't be using antidepressants as a first-line therapy for mild depression; and (b) there's increasing evidence that using antidepressants longer than twelve months is harmful and that we really should be getting people off antidepressants long term. That's pretty radical as well. But it's the sort of statement that can happen from a thorough review of mainstream literature. So in this way I'm more optimistic than David. David says, you know, that the literature is so corrupt. I agree it's pretty corrupt, especially the short-term literature. But you can tease out these long-term studies, even with all the bias, and you see a different picture. So there is some science there that you can, I think, use as a guide to a different way.

It's called The Foundation for Excellence in Mental Healthcare. They will be putting up a website soon. It's hoping to raise quite a bit of money.

QUESTIONER THREE: Yes, as a psychiatric survivor myself, time and time again going to the urgent psychiatric care facility and refusing medication while I'm in a manic state with no physical threat to anyone, I am not given the choice. And then when I refuse to take antipsychotic medication, I then have to go to court where I get placed on a court order where they will force me with injections and whatnot. And I want to know to whom would I turn to find an advocate for myself and other peers? I know this is not uncommon and these medications make me very violent, give me a lot of physical and mental distress and make me far worse. And I was wondering if there are any kinds of campaigns that are going on to help fight the forcing of antipsychotic medication, once we are in these places.

MR. WHITAKER: Yes. Here's what I think the only real answer can be to that. In essence, you've got to make this information known that if you have a person who is in a manic episode or psychotic episode; you're probably going to have to have a safe environment of some sort. Again, this is what Soteria did. If you handle it right, you can create safe spaces such as the Soteria-created safe space. But you do have to create safe spaces. That's not in an emergency room today, unfortunately. The only thing I can say is that it is a challenge as you have to rebuild the system. When that person enters into that sort of extreme psychiatric distress state, you've got to have this long-term knowledge, this long-term perspective, and then you've got to put some effort in—as Western Lapland in Finland does—to create that safe space that will help a person get through that problem without the medication. Or at least give them a chance to do so. And then if at some point it seems like the medication will help, use the medication. But you need to build a safe space. It would be good to listen to people as well, such as your experience is that the drugs make you violent. It would be nice if they would listen to that, I think. All right. Thanks very much.

MODERATOR (Dr. O'Donohue): We will end there. You know, Bob's doing great work, very courageous work, getting hassled sometimes by it. Since we're all mental health professionals, we know the power of positive affirmation. I think you need a little Post-it on your bathroom mirror saying: I'm not as bad as a dictator killing hundreds of thousands of people. So you can keep it up. Thanks.

# References

Andreasen, N. (2005). Longitudinal changes in neurocognition during the first decade of schizophrenic illness. *International Congress of Schizophrenic Research, 348.*

Babyak, M. (2000). Exercise treatment for major depression. *Psychosomatic Medicine, 62,* 633-638.

Baldessarini, R. (1995). Risks and implications of interrupting maintenance of psychotropic drug therapy. *Psychotherapy and Psychosomatics, 63,* 137-141.

Cole, J. (1964). Therapeutic efficacy of antidepressant drugs. *Journal of the American Medical Association, 190,* 448-455.

Coryell, W. (1995). Characteristics and significance of untreated major depressive disorder. *American Journal of Psychiatry, 152,* 1124-1129.

Dewa, C. (2003). Pattern of antidepressant use and duration of depression-related absence from work. *British Journal of Psychiatry, 183,* 507-513.

Fava, G. (1994). Do antidepressants and anxiety drugs increase chronicity in affective disorders? *Psychotherapy and Psychsomatics, 61,* 125-131.

Goldberg, D. (1998). The effects of detection and treatment of major depression in primary care. *British Journal of General Practice, 48,* 1840-1844.

Goodwin, F, (1990). *Manic depressive illness.* New York: Oxford University Press.

Harrow, M. (2007). Factors involved in outcome and recovery in schizophrenia patients not on antipsychotic medications. *Journal of Nervous and Mental Disease, 195,* 406-414.

Hyman, S. (1996). Initiation and adaptation: A paradigm for understanding psychotropic drug action. *American Journal of Psychiatry, 153,* 151-161.

Kendler, K. (2005). As quoted by R. Whitaker, *Anatomy of an epidemic,* New York: Crown; pp. 78-79.

Kline, N. (1964). The practical management of depression. *Journal of the American Medical Association, 190,* 122-130.

Lundquist, G. (1945). Prognosis and course of manic-depressive psychosis. *Acta Psychiatry and Neurology,* Supp. 35, 7-93.

Moncrieff, J. (2000). Trends in sickness benefits in Great Britain and the contribution of mental disorders. *Journal of Public Health Medicine, 22,* 59-67.

Pigott, E. (2010). Efficacy and effectiveness of antidepressants. *Psychotherapy and Psychosomatics, 79,* 267-279.

Shorter, E. (1997). *A history of psychiatry.* New York: Wiley.

Seikkula, J. (2006). Five year experience of first-episode of nonaffective psychosis in open-dialogue approach. *Psychotherapy Research, 16,* 214-228.

Silverman, C. (1968). *The epidemiology of depression.* Baltimore: Johns Hopkins Press.

Social Security Administration (2008). *Annual statistical reports on SSDI and SSI, 1987-2008.*

Stip, E. (2002). "Happy birthday neuroleptics!" *European Psychiatry, 17,* 115-119.

Thatcher, D. (1999). *Mental health: A report of the Surgeon General.* Washington, DC: U.S. Department of Health and Human Services.

Thoriacius, S. (2010). Increased incidence of disability due to mental and behavioural disorders in Iceland, 1990-2007. *Journal of Mental Health, 19,* 176-183.

Tsuang, M. (1979). Long-term outcome if major psychoses. *Archives of General Psychiatry, 36,* 1295-1301.

Van Scheyen, J.D. (1973). Recurrent vital depressions. *Psychiatra, Neurologia, Neurochirurgia, 76,* 93-112.

Viguera, A. (1998). Discontinuing antidepressant treatment in major depression. *Harvard Review of Psychiatry, 5,* 293-305.

Viguera, A. (1997). "Clinical risk following abrupt and gradual withdrawal of maintenance neuroleptic treatment," *Archives of General Psychiatry,* 54, 49-55.

Weel-Baumgarten, E. (2000). Treatment of depression related to recurrence. *Journal of Clinical Psychiatry and Therapeutics, 25,* 61-66.

Whitaker, R. (2010). *Anatomy of an Epidemic.* New York: Crown.

Zarate, C. (2000). Functional impairment and cognition in bipolar disorder. *Psychiatric Quarterly, 71,* 309-329.

Chapter 7

# The Behavioral Care Training Paradigm for the Future

*Ronald O'Donnell. Ph.D.*

Traditional doctoral training in behavioral health, the Ph.D. or Psy.D., represents a significant investment in both time and money. The time required to earn a doctorate and begin practice is seven to eight years. The dissertation typically requires 24 credit hours and at least one year to complete. Student loans can run up to $150,000. A full-year of internship is required, yet due to a current crisis in funding these expensive programs up to 25% of all eligible internship applicants are unable to be placed each year and face the prospect of a one-year wait until the next application cycle. Many doctoral students are interested in careers as practicing psychologists, not academic psychologists. For these students, many of the curriculum courses and the dissertation are not relevant to their long-term career goals. In sum, prospective students interested in an applied clinical doctorate must conduct a serious cost-benefit analysis. Are the rewards, both professionally and financially, of a traditional doctoral degree in behavioral health commensurate with this huge investment? Will the mortgage-size loan that they accrue be offset by long-term salary and benefits?

In terms of career choices, psychologists rank 59 of the top 100 (http://www.jobsrated.com). These ratings are based upon job satisfaction, salary, recognition, stress and related factors. Professions that ranked ahead of psychologists included typists, insurance underwriters, parole officers, and sociologists. These are all worthy professions, but in comparison suggest that psychology has fallen over time in terms of esteem among the public and other professionals. The typical psychologist's salary in the United States is about $82,386. From a return on investment perspective, careers such as surgeon, physician, chief executive, lawyer, and dentist, offer significantly greater average salary and often less investment. In fact, psychologists are the lowest paid doctoral health profession, paid less than pharmacists, podiatrists, optometrists, nurse practitioners, and dentists.

A career as a psychologist was a both an esteemed and lucrative profession decades ago. Nicholas Cummings has noted that other professions, such as dentistry, had similar declines. The profession of dentistry had a crisis in not keeping up with the income of other doctoral professions. They were having problems marketing. However, their professional association took effective steps to reverse this decline. A visit to the modern dentist office includes promotion of many products and services that are not covered or covered in full by major insurance plan benefits. Most importantly, there is a demand by consumers for these new services. Can the profession of doctoral behavioral health providers engineer a similar turnaround, or is it too late?

Another major problem for doctoral clinicians is the glut of psychotherapists. More and more master's degree psychotherapists are graduating and entering the workforce. These include masters in social work, counseling, marital and family therapy, and rehabilitation. In particular, doctoral psychology programs are often the worst culprit, graduating many master's level clinicians who often have a burden trying to practice because of licensure problems. Now, if there was a demand for more psychotherapists, this would be a great thing. But just the opposite is true. Recent studies show decreased use of psychotherapy services across the country, fewer people seeking individual psychotherapy for behavioral problems. The number of patients seeking traditional psychotherapy is declining as more patients turn to medication for relief of behavioral problems (Olfson, 2009).

To add insult to injury, health plans have driven reimbursement rates for doctoral clinicians to the master's level rates. To the public, there is no clear differentiation between a master's level and doctoral level psychotherapists. There is no consumer backlash as health plans effectively steer patients to master's level clinicians and away from doctoral clinicians based on reimbursement. Many clinicians have responded by attempting to market themselves to patients willing to pay out-of-pocket for psychotherapy. However, the pool of patients with the financial means to afford out-of-pocket psychotherapy fees is finite, and not large.

From the perspective of an economist, it is clear that the demand for psychotherapy services is not as great as supply. There are many more therapists trying to engage a dwindling supply of patients. It's common for psychotherapists to blame health plans and managed care for this gap between supply and demand. Many psychotherapists were elated as healthcare parity laws were passed and awaited with great anticipation new patients and revenue streams. But what has happened? Fewer patients, not more, are pursuing psychotherapy. The increase in psychotherapy utilization related to parity laws has been negligible for the average practicing clinician. The movement to increase out of pocket expenses for all healthcare, not just psychotherapy, is but one contributor to this trend. Co-pays in excess of $50 and as high as $100 per session are not unheard of. However, the other likely reason is diminished confidence in the consumer on the value of psychotherapy.

The key question is: can the profession of doctoral behavioral clinicians, such as psychologists, recover from this long and steep decline? The proposition of this chapter is a resounding yes. There are emerging needs that will require specialized behavioral interventions and management skills driven by health-care reform. However, traditional doctoral training programs are not preparing graduates for the needs of the 21st century healthcare system. Professional and accreditation associations for psychologists have continued to commit serious "blunders" that promulgate the training program shortcomings across the entire psychologist profession (Cummings and O'Donohue, 2008). The premise of this chapter is that a new doctoral degree, the Doctor of Behavioral Health (DBH), is a model for "unblundering" doctoral training in order to offer our profession the opportunity to reverse the current free fall in both public esteem and reimbursement.

## Healthcare Reform and Opportunity for Doctoral Behavioral Clinicians

Healthcare reform is an evolving process. The recent healthcare reform legislation is but one step in this evolution, albeit a major one. Details of what final form and shape the current healthcare reform will take are still emerging. However, some key changes are very clear and will have a tremendous impact on healthcare delivery. Cost control is a key driver for health-care reform. Improved prevention and treatment of chronic disease is another key component based on the assumption that this will lead to both improved health outcomes and decreased cost of care.

The concept of integrated care is sweeping the nation with new funding, pilot projects, and training and consultation programs. If you attended any major behavioral health conference five years ago you would be hard pressed to encounter more than a handful of people going attending the integrated care seminars. Now these conference rooms are packed. Across the country there's a huge focus on integrated care. Of course, the main reason for integrated care is trying to improve the treatment of chronic disease, to improve prevention, and disease management.

Integrated care is but one of several major changes speeding from national to local implementation. Among the most significant in payment reform designed to move from the current fee for service reimbursement model to capitation. Of course, after the fiasco of poorly managed capitation in the 1990s the word "capitation" has been replaced with the more respectable sounding "accountable care organization". Significant lobbying for payment reform to steer funds toward primary care physicians and disease prevention is now in motion. There is a movement towards improved healthcare information technology from electronic medical records, to predictive modeling claims database programs, to internet-based behavior change programs. There is an increased focus on evidence-based practice and comparative effectiveness research with the goal of identifying best practices. Quality improvement programs are increasingly incorporating financial incentives (and penalties) for key healthcare delivery process and outcome measurements. These initiatives are designed to reform healthcare in order to improve cost control. This is the area of opportunity for our profession.

First, there is a crisis in primary care. Primary care physicians are in shorter supply and trends in medical school specialization point to that problem increasing. PCP's do not receive significant training in behavioral case identification, assessment, and intervention. They routinely use medications as the first-line and only approach for behavioral problems. Their exposure to evidence-based behavioral interventions is often limited to studies by pharmaceutical companies. Primary care physicians are under-armed and overwhelmed. They do not have the time, resource, energy, education, or know-how to treat the patients coming through their door about behavioral conditions. The first opportunity is for doctoral behavioral clinicians to join primary care medical teams and help to address this crisis.

Chronic medical and behavioral conditions frequently co-occur and the cost of care for these patients is higher than for those with a single chronic condition. The cost of these cases is twice as high as cases with a chronic medical condition only (Kathol et al., 2005). This higher cost is not simply related to increased behavioral health utilization. It's not because these patients are relying upon antidepressant medications or frequently visiting their psychotherapist. Instead, the higher costs are driven by medical utilization, medical procedures, hospitalizations, labs, imaging, and physician visits. Chronic disease management for both medical and behavioral conditions relies on behavior change, especially for lifestyle problems such as poor nutrition, overeating and obesity, lack of physical activity and cigarette smoking. The second opportunity is for psychologists to take the lead in designing, conducting, and evaluating disease management programs.

Physical symptoms overlap with behavioral conditions, making it difficult for physicians to identify stress and behavioral problems underlying symptom presentation. Nicholas Cummings seminal work on somatizers identified patients with medically unexplained multiple physical symptoms were going to their physician or their nurse for relief. Research shows 60–70% of all physician visits are for physical symptoms with no medical etiology (Fries et al., 1993). Most patients with anxiety and depression present with physical symptoms. They don't talk about their mood being down or being anxious or worried. They talk about physical symptoms that are bothering them. Most physicians treat the symptom by offering medication for the symptoms rather than identifying and treating the underlying issue: stress, conflict, family problems driving those physical symptoms.

Somatizers are a well-researched group. The cost for these patients is 6 to 14 times higher than non-somatizer patients. They experience high impairments in terms of their work and their family life. Their behavioral stress problems are typically overlooked and not treated by physicians (Katon et al., 1991; Smith et al., 1986). These patients often begin a long search for medical disease and a medical solution to their problems. Research has demonstrated that brief, behavioral interventions such as individual psychotherapy or stress management group treatment effectively reduce symptoms and decrease medical cost. Yet these studies have not been widely adopted in primary care, resulting in a wasted opportunity for our profession to both improve patient care and reduce excessive medical utilization and cost. The ability to recognize somatizers and provide efficient and effective interventions represents the third opportunity for psychologists.

It's essential to stay attuned to the healthcare concerns of a key stakeholder: large employers. Employers contract with highly reimbursed consultants to advise them about how to better manage their workforce. In recent years, there has been a spotlight on the problem of the high cost they're paying for behavioral and medical chronic conditions. The costs of lost productivity absenteeism, presenteeism (people going to work and just not really being engaged in their work), and disability claims due to chronic disease is tremendous. The costs associated with lost productivity and disability is three times the cost of medical claims alone for those patients (Loeppke et al., 2007). In effect, employers are paying for employee healthcare twice. First, they support our health insurance premiums, and second, they are paying for lost productivity and disability due to chronic disease. And they can quantify this. The industry now relies on cost calculators based on algorithms that can project the impact of conditions such as depression based on workforce type and size.

Employers are desperate for solutions to the high cost of chronic illness. They have utilized Employee Assistance Programs (EAPs) for decades and have recently turned towards integrating EAP practice with primary care. In addition, employers have partnered with health plans and associated vendors using expensive disease management programs. These companies utilize health plan claims data in order to develop sophisticated algorithms to identify high-risk, high-cost patients. These companies employ medical and behavioral clinicians who then outreach these patients by mail and phone to offer disease management, health coaching, and prevention. These programs are well designed and combine evidence-based practice with sophisticated health information technology. The problem with these programs is abysmal patient engagement. Enrollment, continuation, and completion of these programs is often less than ten percent of the target population. It's not surprising that when an unknown clinician makes a cold call to a patient identified via health plan claims data and asks to speak about their most personal health problems, the patient response is often negative. Typical patient questions include: "Who are you? How did you get my information? Where are you calling from?" It should not be surprising that patients decline these programs.

As a result of low engagement, these disease management programs fail to deliver on promised return on investment (ROI). If you target 1000 patients for interventions, but only 100 are enrolled, you're not going to achieve cost savings. For patients who do engage, these programs can be very successful. They will offer significant benefits for the 100 or so patients who enroll and complete the program. The remaining 900 prospective enrollees do not benefit from the program, and will offset any potential cost-savings for the 100 patients enrolled in the program. The problem of failure to deliver on promised ROI is now widely recognized by employers. One approach with promise is to structure these programs with workplace incentives or consequences that reward participation and sometimes penalize non-participation. Typical incentives include reduced medical premiums or small payments for completion of specific health programs. However, one approach that has not been widely utilized is integrated care. A behavioral clinician could contract with employers to work with these employees in coordination with their primary care physician. Nicholas Cummings' work on outlier outreach disease management programs demonstrated that when the behavioral clinician makes a cold call from the primary care office as a member of the primary care team, participation exceeds 90%. Patients trust their primary care physician. The ability of doctoral behavioral clinicians to bridge the gap between the workplace and primary care with specialized population-based interventions to address the impact of chronic illness on workplace productivity is the fourth opportunity for doctoral behavioral clinicians.

Another problem that is receiving deserved attention is the overuse of pharmacological treatments as a first line intervention for behavioral conditions. The problems are multifaceted. Pharmacology is often the sole line of treatment. When a medication is not effective, a typical response is to try an alternative medication. When alternatives are exhausted, medication combinations or cocktails are offered. First, as outlined in other chapters in this volume, the evidence base for the effectiveness of pharmacological treatment for behavioral conditions is under increased criticism. An emerging consensus is that pharmacological treatment is not effective for many behavioral interventions, and alternative behavioral interventions are more clinically effective and cost-effective. Second, even when appropriate medications are prescribed they are prescribed at dosages too low to be clinically effective based on research findings (Simon, 2002). Third, a high percentage of patients discontinue medications prematurely. Side effects are common and a significant reason for discontinuation. Studies that compare physician and patient ratings of medication side-effects show a gap between physician and patient perspectives. Patients rate medication side-effects as a significant problem, while physician ratings show much lower recognition of how problematic side-effects are for their patients (Hu et al., 2004). Fourth, in the popular press and patient community we are seeing a backlash against the promise of pharmacological treatment. Fifth, and last of all, patients, when they're polled, would prefer psychotherapy over pharmacological treatment if it was available to them (Van Schaik et al., 2004). In summary, first line pharmacological treatment is often ineffective, frequently discontinued by patients; and patients are interested in non-pharmacological alternatives. The prospect of offering psychotherapy as a first line intervention rather than medications in primary care represents the fifth key opportunity for doctoral behavioral providers.

Health information technology is another key component of healthcare reform with implications for behavioral health. Initiatives such as electronic medical records and collection and analysis of health information data are common examples. The trend of greatest significance to behavioral health is the emerging field behavioral ehealth. Examples include using e-mail, instant messaging, chat rooms, or distance medicine using videoconferencing. Of perhaps greater interest is the emergence of internet-based behavior change programs. In these programs, patients use interactive online learning tools to learn how to effectively self-manage their chronic conditions.

Behavioral ehealth programs are now widely available Europe and Australia, and are emerging to prominence in the United States. Research using randomized controlled studies now demonstrates that online cognitive-behavioral therapy-based self-help programs are as effective as in-person treatment for conditions such as depression, anxiety, substance abuse, and PTSD (Kay-Lambkin et al., 2009; Knaevelsrud and Maercker 2007; MacKinnnon et al., 2007; Reger and Gahm, 2009). It's important to note that simply supplying a patient the URL for a web-based behavior change program is not sufficient. There must be a clinician involved in-person with the patient, helping to guide them on use these tools and evaluate their progress. Without a clinician and some face-to-face contact, these internet-based programs are ineffective. Behavioral ehealth is best viewed as an adjunct to in-person treatment.

In addition, ehealth interventions deliver efficiencies and help move treatment from the office to the patient's home. In terms of efficiency, research shows savings of 50–80% of therapist time compared to in-person treatment by using these web-based behavioral change tools (Marks and Cavanagh 2009). This makes intuitive sense. For example, the time a cognitive-behavioral therapist spends in-person explaining concepts such as self-monitoring and thought-change techniques could be significantly reduced with the patient completing such introductory, educational activities online at home. The patient goes home with your direction, learns and practices these techniques, and receives automated feedback on their progress. The next session the patient reviews his or her progress in your session. The potential for doctoral behavioral clinicians to utilize behavioral ehealth interventions to both improve treatment outcome and increase efficiency represent the sixth opportunity for our profession.

Accountability is the final key component of healthcare reform, and perhaps the most important. The term "accountable care organization" refers to a model of healthcare delivery in which payment is provided in a lump sum, commonly called capitation, for a defined patient population. It is the responsibility of the organization to provide necessary care and to demonstrate that specific healthcare process and outcome criteria are achieved or met. In many cases there are financial incentives based on measures to which the organization are held accountable. In the accountable care organization, the leadership and clinicians must partner to provide value-based services that are both clinically and cost-effective. They have their services measured routinely. In addition, a key focus of healthcare incentives will be improved management of chronic illness as measured by condition-specific process and outcome measures. Leaders and clinicians who can develop treatment programs that demonstrate improved clinical outcome and cost-effectiveness will go to the front of the line. This represents the seventh key opportunity for doctoral behavioral clinicians. We have proven interventions that result in improved clinical outcome, high patient satisfaction, and a reduction in the excess cost associated with overuse of unnecessary medical services.

Finally, if given a choice, most patients would prefer to receive behavioral treatment in their primary care office, not via referral to a specialty care office or clinic. Research shows that when offered a referral from their physician to see a behavioral specialist, the vast majority do not even attend a single appointment. The reasons are multifaceted. Patients have great trust in their family physician relative to other professions. Conversely, patients often have low confidence in the ability of behavioral specialists to effectively treat their conditions. So, patients continue to receive referrals from their physician, fail to follow-up, and focus on the medical healthcare system to address their behavioral conditions. Conversely, if you offer treatment right there in the primary care physician's office, 80% plus will engage. From a healthcare economics perspective, this represents the eighth key opportunity for doctoral clinicians. The traditional specialty private practice model of psychotherapy is faced with an oversupply of psychotherapists and a decreasing demand from patients. In primary care, you have a deficit of appropriately trained behavioral clinicians and an oversupply of patients who are currently under-identified and undertreated. Healthcare reform dollars are increasing in the integrated care arena, and remain flat in specialty behavioral health.

# The Unmet Educational Need

The good news is that the health-care market seems to be looking for things that doctoral behavioral clinicians are perfectly tailored for. The eight opportunities outlined above are driven by the marketplace and are in play for the right type of provider to meet these needs. The bad news is: many of the skills essential to take advantage of these opportunities are not typically offered in traditional doctoral degree programs. Instead, doctoral training continues to include many courses that are irrelevant to the future of applied clinical practice. In an effort to support the "scientist-practitioner", multiple courses in statistics and research design are required. The dissertation is based on a model of peer-reviewed academic research. These are excellent courses for a psychologist interested in a career in academia. However, for the average clinical psychologist who plans to practice in applied settings, these are courses that will have no relevance and never be used again upon graduation. Worse yet, the types of research design including measurement and statistical analysis that are commonly used in modern healthcare are not offered in traditional programs. Quality improvement models, HEDIS measures (Healthcare Effectiveness Data and Information Set), return on investment, and medical cost offset are absent from traditional program curriculum.

Psychotherapy training in traditional programs is based on private practice or specialty clinic models in which longer term psychotherapy using the traditional fifty-minute hour reigns supreme. Taking a course in the history and systems of psychotherapy is certainly interesting, but not relevant to the applied doctoral clinician. Internship training is based on an outmoded and inefficient model that will soon be supplanted by more innovative approaches to training. Training is typically classroom-based, followed by a full-year internship and then a full-year post-doctoral position. The excellent book *The Innovators Prescription* (Christensen et al. 2009) predicts that the model for clinical training in the future will make coursework and clinical work *simultaneous* so that students can immediately apply what they learn in clinical settings. Otherwise, knowledge that is learned in a classroom setting will not transfer to patients that are seen one, two or even three years after that class is completed.

As a consequence of the many irrelevant courses that traditional doctoral programs require, it is not unusual for a Ph.D. or Psy.D to require upwards of 110–120 credit hours to complete the degree. The dissertation alone requires students to take 24 credit hours of coursework. This makes a doctoral degree a very expensive proposition. Other professions, such as nursing, have moved to offering applied clinical doctorates that only require 84 credit hours for graduation. The curriculum of these applied doctoral degree programs are flexible and based on the needs of the healthcare market. As prospective students do the math and calculate the cost-benefit ratio for a Ph.D. or Psy.D versus other alternatives, it is likely new applied doctoral degrees will begin to have a clear advantage.

## Professional Blunders

The anti-business, anti-healthcare agenda noted by Nicholas Cummings is alive and well in our profession. Cummings and O'Donohue (2008) conclude that most behavioral clinicians are economic illiterates. As a profession, we are simply not good at understanding how healthcare economics, healthcare financing, and emerging models for paid performance; performance incentives are about to reshape healthcare as we know it. A typical refrain of practicing psychologists is to bemoan the latest fee reduction for their insurance panel and cry for fee increases based on the value of the doctoral degree. Unfortunately for them, fees are determined by economic forces in the market, not by social values. Psychologists continue to clamor for more money for behavioral health and attack payers such as health plans and managed care companies. One has to question the soundness of a strategy that relies on continued attacks against those who are in charge of reimbursement in healthcare. In spite of occasional successes against health plans and managed care companies, the landscape of reimbursement for doctoral clinicians remains unchanged.

In addition, we continue to pride ourselves as being a profession separate from and literally outside of medicine. The private practice model continues to be the predominant model in our profession. Unfortunately, from the perspective of healthcare economics, this is the last place you would want to be. Healthcare GDP has increased from 7 to 15% of our budget from 1970 to 2009 (Frank et al., 2009). Mental healthcare spending has been relatively flat during that same time period, at less than 1%. In which healthcare system do you want to work? One with significant and continued increases in spending over the past 40 years, or one that has been in decline and has remained flat for decades?

The other area in which our profession continues to operate in attack mode (or denial) is accountability. In medicine and soon psychotherapy, there will be routine requirements to measure clinical processes and outcomes, as well as cost-effectiveness. Psychologists are often the loudest to complain that psychotherapy work cannot be effectively measured. In launching outcomes management programs, it is often the psychologists who attack the use of empirically supported outcome measures. Typical refrains include: "We can't really measure all the dimensions of my patients because they're so complex, they're so unique. That measure wouldn't work for my practice. We aren't quite at the stage yet we can measure outcome empirically with valid measures." For a profession founded upon principles of behavioral and psychological assessment, these responses seem indefensible.

Instead, the root of the concern is being accountable. Accountability means that you will be compared to your peer clinicians on the basis of objective performance measures. Further, these measures will be used in incentive programs and made public. On the plus side, evidence shows that, in aggregate, psychotherapy is effective and that most clinicians help the majority of patients. On the downside, it's also clear that there exists significant variability in psychologist effectiveness, with some being significantly better than others in both the magnitude of their clinical effect size and their efficiency, the ability of their patients to demonstrate significant improvement in shorter periods of time. The prospect of accountability is simply terrifying to many clinicians for this reason.

This leads to a similar blunder: the attack on making healthcare costs part of the dialog on behavioral health and psychotherapy. A common refrain among psychologists is that the benefits of psychotherapy should be accepted at face value without concern for cost-effectiveness, let alone cost savings. However, healthcare is a business driven by economics. Every health plan is focused on return on investment and searching for ways to decrease inappropriate utilization and cost. This is an area that psychologists should excel in, given their backgrounds in both research on program evaluation and statistical analysis. Unfortunately, it is an arena largely occupied by nurses and physicians, actuaries and finance managers. Further, the research on medical cost offset related to behavioral interventions is not well understood by nurses, physicians and actuaries and begs for an insightful psychologist to help design, implement and evaluate such programs.

Next, let's look at credentialing for doctoral behavioral clinicians. The American Psychological Association has two competing constituencies: academics and clinicians. Nicholas Cummings and members of the National Alliance of Practicing Professional Psychologists have shared stories of psychologists being their own worst enemy. Often academic psychologists with no significant clinical experience are the ones blocking progressive initiatives such as psychologist prescribing privileges, in spite of the majority of applied, practicing psychologists endorsing them. Nearly every other health profession has an established credentialing body that is operated by applied clinicians who are making a living doing what they are responsible for credentialing. Our profession is a glaring exception.

A related blunder is a lack of innovative, forward-thinking leadership. The problem is twofold. First, valuable time and resources are exhausted fighting for ways to preserve historical patterns of practice rather than leading towards new models that will match the needs of 21st century healthcare reform. Second, the pace of change within the American Psychological Association is glacial. Endless committees spend years debating issues, years turn into decades, and the profession remains frozen. Contrast this with leadership in the dental profession, who quickly recognized a decline in professional status and income and took dramatic steps in short order to effectively address them. Healthcare reform is happening now and opportunities will not wait for committee decisions. Look at the field of nursing. They are prepared to replace primary care clinicians. Perhaps unbeknownst to psychologists, they are also preparing to replace our profession in delivering behavioral care in primary care settings. The College of Nursing and Health Innovation here at Arizona State University is representative. They already have clinical tracks in child and adolescent behavioral problems. Nurses have training in healthcare management and program evaluation that is based on our evolving healthcare system, and are using this knowledge and training to move into leadership positions throughout the healthcare system. The healthcare market is not going to wait for psychologists to carefully weigh in on the shape of new initiatives. Successful professional associations are characterized by a vision that retains a focus on improving patient care, but also is responsive to the emerging market demands and working quickly and effectively to improve the prestige and financial status of their members. Contrast this to the American Psychological Association. This represents a continued major blunder.

How do you measure proficiency currently for most doctoral training programs and for doctoral behavioral clinicians? We use course grades, number of hours of supervision, ratings from supervisors, a national examination for psychologists, and CEU certificates. State licensure requirements for clinical psychologists are largely based on the APA accreditation standards (APA, 2007) as well as the Association of State and Provincial Psychology Boards (ASPPB, 2010). The national exam for psychologists, the EPPP, is based on many items that, while relevant for academic researchers, are not for applied doctoral clinicians (O'Donohue and Buchannan, 2003). What do all of these approaches have in common? They do not include objective data based on the clinicians work with patients! Measures of patient processes, outcomes, and treatment alliance that are based on patient reports are not typically used to evaluate performance. Now, if you pick a surgeon out for a procedure you want to have done, my guess is you're looking for evidence such as how many procedures he or she has completed. What has their outcome been? Are their patient satisfaction survey results available? These are objective outcome measures. How many psychologists use these types of metrics to help the public evaluate their potential services? Instead, proxies for clinical performance, such as hours of supervision and CEUs, become institutionalized in state boards of psychology to demonstrate competency.

The final area in which the American Psychological Association continues to blunder is in the area of telemedicine or ehealth. In medicine, telemedicine is used to train clinicians. Diagnosis is made by videoconference examinations. A physician in California can help diagnose and treat a patient in Florida. Surgery can be conducted via video. In contrast, our profession does not recognize videoconferencing for supervision. Again, other professions embrace and utilize these innovative new technologies, while we either ignore them, at best, or strongly resist and fight them, at worst. The APA, ASPPB and individual states are grappling with challenges such as portability of licensure, distance learning, telehealth, ehealth, and supervision requirements (DeMers et al., 2008).

The traditional models of training doctoral level behavioral care providers—primarily clinical psychologists—are increasingly criticized for these blunders. Significant challenges from within and outside of the APA and ASPPB are raising controversy and gaining ground. The National Alliance of Professional Psychology Providers (NAPPP) was formed in 2006 as a professional organization for practicing psychologists solely dedicated to the advocacy of practicing doctoral clinicians. The Association for Psychological Science (APS) announced a new accreditation system for clinical science, the Psychological Clinical Science Accreditation System (PCSAS) with a series of media releases highly critical of the APA and psychologists for not incorporating empirically supported research into clinical practice. In response to these criticisms, the APA has moved to make initial, incremental changes such as defining psychology as part of rather than separate from the healthcare system, and promoting integrated care as a career path for psychologists. New standards for professional competency assessment were recently established (APA 2006). The APA and ASPPB have recommended dropping the requirement of a post-doctoral training and replaced it with two years of combined internship and internship experience. These are positive steps, but they are incremental and fall far short of other professions that have reacted quickly and effectively to the emerging demands of 21st century healthcare reform.

## Unblundering: The Doctor of Behavioral Health

The premise of this chapter is that radical reform in educating and training is needed to prepare a new workforce of *applied, doctoral level* behavioral care providers specializing in integrated care. The new Doctor of Behavioral Health degree program at Arizona State University will serve as a case study to highlight solutions to the continued blunders of traditional training, association leadership, and accreditation. The recommendations for reform include:

- A new applied, professional doctorate degree in integrated behavioral health
- A new professional accreditation body for the degree
- A flexible course curriculum that eliminates courses irrelevant to practicing clinicians and adds courses essential to meet the demands of healthcare reform (which will be continual)
- Eliminate the dissertation and replace it with a research project that focuses on the skills needed to demonstrate cost-effectiveness in healthcare
- Upgrade master's level licensed clinicians for enrollment in order to deliver more doctoral level integrated care clinicians in medical settings
- Approve distance learning and distance supervision for internship training
- Incorporate ehealth and telemedicine into practice training

- Adopt the competency model recommended by the APA Task Force (APA, 2006)
- Create a new national examination specific to competencies of applied practitioners

In 2008, Nicholas Cummings, in collaboration with leadership in Arizona State University, developed the Doctor of Behavioral Health (DBH) program. The DBH is a new doctoral degree in behavioral health designed to train behavioral clinicians to provide integrated care in medical settings. The program is based on models of professional training and credentialing typical of most other healthcare professions. The DBH program reform is *radical* in that it: (1) is founded on a knowledge base that incorporates clinical skills in integrated care, medical literacy, healthcare economics, and entrepreneurship; (2) relies on a small core, non-tenured faculty complimented with adjunct faculty and clinical supervisors who are practicing clinicians; (3) provides hands-on internship experience in primary care and related settings; (4) systematically collects individual and program outcome data in order to evaluate competency; (5) embraces the mission of producing behavioral care providers who have the ability to produce and document medical cost-offset in their clinical practice, and; (6) has received provisional accreditation by a new entity, the National Institute of Behavioral Health Quality, formed under the auspices of the National Alliance of Professional Psychology Providers.

The DBH is *traditional* in that it is designed to: (1) meet the requirements for accreditation as a program of psychology by the APA; (2) meet key guidelines on internship experience endorsed by the ASPPB, and; (3) meet anticipated requirements for doctoral licensure as APA and ASPPB recommendations are adopted by state licensing boards. The DBH program is *progressive* in that it: (1) has already incorporated a comprehensive competency assessment program; (2) replaces the dissertation with a rigorous, yet relevant research project; (3) uses distance learning in order to make courses and supervision available to students around the world, and; (4) incorporates innovative ehealth approaches as an adjunct to treatment.

The program requires 84 credit hours for completion, 30 of which are credited from the clinicians' master's degree program. The remaining 54 credit hours include 10 core courses, 4 elective courses, a culminating research project, and internship. The internship program begins in the second semester of the program and is based on a sequential, stage-based training with students completing an average of two, eight-hour days per week in each semester for a total of 400 hours of internship experience. The program may be completed in 18 months in an accelerated program that includes summer sessions.

The DBH core faculty is small and comprised of clinical psychologists with experience in integrated care as practitioners. Adjunct faculty members are typically contracted psychologists with excellent teaching skills and full-time professional experience in the area in which they are teaching. The adjunct faculty all make a living doing what they are teaching. In addition, the faculty includes representatives by other healthcare graduate programs in the university, such as nursing, a doctoral health and wellness program, a behavioral health research department, the school of business healthcare administration, and public health.

## The Curriculum

### *The Macro-curriculum*

Medical literacy courses are designed to prepare the behavioral clinicians with a broad survey of clinical medicine and pathophysiology, psychopharmacology, and clinical neuropathophysiology. These courses are designed to present a survey of disease etiology, course and progression, medical treatment, and outcome. The objective is for the behavioral clinician to understand and consult with medical providers within a multidisciplinary team setting and converse in the language of these providers.

The integrated behavioral care provider will need a thorough understanding of the healthcare system in order to grasp the implications of healthcare reform, and business entrepreneur skills to be able to respond proactively to pursue career and economic opportunities in the changing healthcare environment (O'Donohue et al., 2009). The DBH course on healthcare systems and economics includes healthcare policy and reform, financing and reimbursement, and quality and accreditation. The behavioral entrepreneurship course includes: (1) personality factors and attitudes that contribute to success; (2) how market forces enhance or limit success; (3) steps and resources needed for a "start-up" company; (4) venture capital and investment; (5) compensation; (6) business law and regulation; (7) how to write, present, implement and evaluate a business plan, and; (8) exit strategy. The objective is to increase the ability of the behavioral care provider to demonstrate value-added to healthcare payers as a means of expanding his or her economic base.

A core course in population health management reviews principles of disease management programs, examples from the industry, and student projects in which they design their own outlier outreach project for a high-risk, high-cost patient population. The course in research design is focused on how healthcare processes and outcomes are measured in medical healthcare settings. Traditional quality improvement study design is incorporated with return on investment analysis. The goal is to prepare DBH clinicians to both utilize existing primary care or hospital quality improvement and return on investment models and introduce their own proposals that are behavioral health specific.

## *The Clinical Curriculum*

The clinical skills necessary for effective delivery of integrated behavioral care are not the same as those necessary for traditional mental health and substance abuse treatment settings. McDaniel et al. (2002) noted that the provider must be a generalist that is responsive to a wide range of medical and behavioral problems for diverse populations across the lifespan. Principles of population-based management and stepped care are essential, yet foreign to most behavioral clinicians (Strosahl, 2005). In addition, the behavioral provider must be able to function as a member of a multidisciplinary medical team, usually headed by a primary care physician, and in consultation with other specialists. The shift from traditional behavioral health into the medical culture, the values, beliefs, norms and behaviors that comprise the medical mindset, are a dramatic challenge since they run directly counter to how traditional psychotherapy is delivered: visits are brief; the therapist is on the floor interacting with the team and ready for a "hallway hand-off" at any time; sessions may be interrupted for crises; verbal and written communication must be concrete, action-oriented, symptom-focused and evidence-based. There is substantial pressure to summarize and distill a large amount of essential information that can be a source of stress that overwhelms the unprepared trainee (Satterfield, 2003).

Strosahl (2005) provides an excellent summary of core domains and practice competencies required for integrated behavioral care. The first domain, clinical practice skills, includes; rapid problem identification and patient engagement, a strengths model, ability to help the client focus on specific problems and functional outcomes, medical literacy, health psychology, preventive health and lifestyle change interventions. The domain of practice management skills includes: effective use of brief sessions, screening and outcomes measurement, time management, knowledge of community-based resources, flexible and creative scheduling and contact strategies (e.g., phone, email), and case management. The consultation skills domain includes; ability to focus on the referral question and provide effective feedback to the medical team, expertise in psychopharmacology in order to effectively consult with prescribers, leading efforts to develop behavioral health clinical pathways, and recommendations that help to reduce physician workload and improve productivity. Documentation skills include: recording the referral question, timely, clear and concise notes on the treatment plan and progress. Team performance skills include: awareness of team roles and functions effectively within the medical culture, frequent rounds on the floor in order to enhance awareness of behavioral services, readily responds to consultation by cell phone, and willing to provide in-service training. Administrative skills include understanding and following policies, procedures and protocols. France et al. (2008) also provide an excellent summary of core knowledge based and applied competencies based on APA Task Force recommendations. The DBH program has incorporated this knowledge and applied competencies into the curriculum and internship.

## The Critical Ingredients: Efficiency and Medical Cost Offset

A distinguishing feature of the DBH clinical curriculum is a clinical training on the Biodyne model of integrated care and psychotherapy described in detail by Cummings and Sayama (1995) and Cummings and Cummings (2000). The model was developed by Nicholas Cummings beginning in the late 1950s in Kaiser Permanente and subsequently refined over the course of five decades in the Hawaii Medicaid Project (Cummings, 2002) and in the training and supervision of hundreds of psychologists in the American Biodyne managed care company. The Biodyne model is seen as critical for two key reasons. First, the model is based on *efficient* delivery of clinical services. Efficiency is achieved largely through the use of therapeutic strategies and techniques designed to effectively manage patient resistance and achieve rapid therapeutic alliance. In addition, the service delivery model focused on clinician productivity and efficiency using group treatment protocols. Second, the Biodyne model has consistently demonstrated what Cummings and associates termed "medical cost offset". Medical cost offset is used to describe how focused, targeted behavioral interventions delivered in primary care lead to reductions in medical cost that are greater than or offset the cost of delivering the behavioral intervention (Cummings, 2002). The reductions in medical cost are due to decreased overuse of medical services such as primary care physician visits, specialist referrals, labs, and imaging. These savings are achieved by the combination of efficient provision of effective psychotherapy plus population-based management of high utilizing patients via telephonic outreach, behavioral interventions and case management. For example, a recent integrated care study by Chaffee et al. (in preparation) reported a 21% reduction in total medical costs in integrated care settings compared to utilization the year prior.

The service delivery model is based on clinician time in the primary care setting consists of: 25% individual appointments; 50% in group disease and population programs, and 25% in group psychotherapy. The group disease programs include conditions such as asthma, diabetes, hypertension, obesity, and fibromyalgia. The psychotherapy groups include phobias, bereavement, borderline personality disorder, depression, schizophrenia, anxiety, and panic. (Cummings & Cummings, 2005). The group culture greatly facilitates treatment progress. Each group program is based on: (1) treatment of the behavioral and medical aspects of each condition; (2) facilitating patient self-management of chronic aspects of their illness, and; (3) prevention of relapse or worsening of outcomes due to poor condition self-management. The group protocols share common characteristics that are interchangeable between specific groups, such as: patient education; pain management; relaxation and stress management; homework assignments; and a self-management component in which patients learn to self-monitor and manage biomedical and behavioral indicators.

The Biodyne model of psychotherapy and service delivery is an *anagram* in that current and emerging evidence-based practice are continuously added to the individual and group protocols into a Biodyne treatment manual. For example, many of the protocols in James and O'Donohue (2008) and O'Donohue et al., (2005) are in use. The manual is designed to be easily modified based on the unique characteristics of the treatment setting. A treatment protocol for depression will be different for American Indians in a reservation in Arizona, for rural patients in a small PCP office in Iowa, or urban Latino patients in downtown Phoenix. The modular formatting of these treatment manual components enables each group protocol to serve different populations with similar treatment needs by inserting or substituting modules, further contributing to efficiency.

## The Culminating Research Project

The DBH program replaces the dissertation with a culminating project that is a scholarly, applied clinical research project. The culminating research project is designed to demonstrate the students' ability to design an integrated behavioral care intervention, including a literature review, appropriate research design and analysis, reporting of results and discussion. Examples of studies include group therapy interventions, population health interventions, and screening projects. In addition, the culminating project includes a business plan component. The study is encouraged to develop a proposal that he or she plans to provide after graduation. The business plan, in effect, is a marketing proposal that the students will use to refine his or her skills in presenting a compelling proposal to payers in healthcare, such as physician groups, hospitals, and health plans. In fact, students are encouraged to develop a business portfolio during their studies that summarizes their performance metrics, such as patient self-reported outcomes, workplace productivity measures, and projected cost-savings or medical cost-offset and return on investment. While the project is completed in the final semester, the student actively develops the project with his advisor and develops the proposal. In this manner, the research project is developed as part of a comprehensive, sequential learning experience.

## The DBH Internship Program

The DBH internship program affords students the opportunity to function as behavioral care providers in a primary care clinics and similar settings. The program is based on a sequential model that includes competency levels tied to the course curriculum progression. In the novice stage, the students learn about the culture of primary care, the role of the behavioral care provider, and the model of targeted, focused behavioral interventions. In the intermediate phase, the student focuses on screening, assessment and treatment of the most common behavioral conditions in primary care, such as depression, anxiety, substance abuse, and somatizers. Students begin focus on co-morbid medical and behavioral chronic conditions and lifestyle interventions designed to enhance health and wellness. In the advanced phase, the student integrates course material on more challenging conditions, such as schizophrenia and psychotic disorders, borderline personality disorders, and suicide prevention. Students also focus on couples and family interventions, and specialization in areas such as pediatrics.

# DBH Internship Program Supervision

The DBH program internship supervision is provided by licensed psychologists who are DBH faculty or contracted with the program. Supervisors are experienced in the Biodyne model, integrated care, and trained in the DBH competency model described below. Students meet in small group supervision for 60 minutes per week. Group size is kept small to facilitate discussion, typically five to eight students. Online students meet in groups with webcams that enable a streaming image of each participant on the computer. Audio recordings of clinician-patient sessions are reviewed routinely during the program, and students are encouraged to use mini-video cameras or cell phone video recording of sessions when possible. The audio and video recordings are reviewed by the group for discussion and feedback. The supervisor is the key liaison between the DBH program and the internship site preceptor for student performance feedback on an as needed basis and during regular student performance evaluations.

# DBH Internship Sites

The DBH program contracts with primary care offices using an affiliation agreement that defines responsibilities of the clinic, the DBH program, and the internship student. Sites vary in size and complexity, from integrated delivery systems to solo practices, from sites serving largely commercial insurance products to Federally Qualified Health Centers. Unlike traditional doctoral training clinics, these sites generally do not have dedicated behavioral clinicians affiliated with the office to provide supervision and oversight. These arrangements simply do not exist today, and this is the gap the DBH program aims to fill. Instead, each internship site identifies a preceptor to oversee each student and serve as liaison with the DBH program. The preceptor ideally is a medical health provider. Responsibilities of the preceptor include orientation of the student to office policy and procedures and the work environment, facilitating introduction of the student to the medical team and support staff, and facilitation of the collection of measures of student performance.

# Competency Assessment

The DBH program is based on a comprehensive model of competency assessment based on a developmentally informed, multi-method and multi-informant process using established evaluation tools. Assessment results are reviewed sequentially in the program in order to obtain formative and summative results matched to training goals. Assessment results are incorporated into supervision in the program and in the internship site, and reviewed with the student advisor over the course of the program. First, a rating scale of integrated care knowledge and applied competencies (Robinson and Reiter, 2007) is used to evaluate student performance. The assessment dimensions are: (1) clinical practice skills; (2) practice management; (3) consultation; (4) documentation; (5) team performance, and; (6) administrative. The ratings are completed by the student as a self-assessment, by the DBH internship supervisor, and by clinicians at the internship site. These forms are administered, collected, analyzed, and reviewed with each student, DBH supervisor, internship preceptor, and advisor near the end of each semester.

Second, an outcomes management program is used to collect and evaluate patient progress based on measures of clinical outcome and treatment alliance. The measures are the Outcome Rating Scale (ORS) and the Session Rating Scale (SRS) developed by Barry Duncan and Scott Miller (Miller et al., 2006). Research has demonstrated that the systematic collection and review of patient outcomes feedback by clinicians during the course of behavioral treatment has positive effects on treatment outcome (Harmon et al., 2007). Reviewing outcomes and alliance in real time allows the clinician to adjust the treatment plan for patients who are deteriorating or not making expected progress in treatment. Research on the ORS and SRS demonstrated that outcomes and treatment alliance feedback resulted in a significant improvement in clinical effectiveness and improved treatment retention (Miller et al., 2006). The DBH program contracted with the company MyOutcomes (www.myoutcomes.com) in order to provide internet access to and real time scoring and feedback of the ORS and SRS. The system automatically tracks and reports patient progress and the students review these results in supervision. In addition, MyOutcomes will generate reports that will summarize effect size and other measures for each student, for each internship site, and for the DBH program in aggregate.

Third, the DBH program has contracted with ProChange Behavior Systems (www.prochange.com), a company founded by James Prochaska, in order to make available to DBH students and their patients a suite of internet-based, patient behavior change computer programs based on gthe Transtheoretical Model of behavior change. The ProChange system uses patient self-assessment based on the patients' stage of change to develop individually tailored behavior change interventions (Prochaska et al., 2008). Patients complete these assessments at monthly intervals and receive individually tailored feedback. These approaches have demonstrated significant improvement for many behavioral conditions, including diet, exercise, stress and depression (Prochaska et al., 2008). The DBH student will assign patients to work on specific ProChange programs outside of sessions as a means of using homework to extend the benefits of treatment. The contract with ProChange will make available program level, aggregate reports for all users. The individual student will need to review and collect individual patient reports manually in order to incorporate this data into treatment planning.

Fourth, the program incorporates measures of clinician productivity and efficiency necessary for calculating medical cost offset. The Biodyne criterion for effectiveness is reduction in patient medical and surgical service utilization from the start of treatment compared to a full year's utilization in a one-year period prior to the start of treatment. Efficiency is measured based on the number of weighted sessions per treatment episode (Cummings, 2002). For example, individual sessions are counted based on the number of minutes of contact, whereas a two-hour group session with one therapist and eight patients is weighted one-fourth of an hour per patient. The cost-effectiveness ratio is the average number of medical services for one year prior to the start of treatment divided by the average medical utilization in the year after treatment initiation plus the number of weighted behavioral treatment sessions for that group of patients (Cummings, 2002).

Fifth, students routinely administer a measure of work productivity, the Work Productivity Activity Impairment Scale (WPAI) (http://www.reillyassociates.net). Employers are increasingly aware of the adverse impact of chronic medical and behavioral conditions on workforce productivity and they are searching for health promotion and disease management programs in an effort to reign in the increasing costs of lost productivity and disability. Internship students administer the WPAI at the beginning of treatment and at six month intervals post treatment initiation. The WPAI data can be used to calculate the dollars saved by employers based on improvements in productivity.

## Credentials

The DBH program limits enrollment to master's level, licensed behavioral clinicians, such as social workers, counselors, and marital and family therapists. The rationale for this criterion is that the DBH, as a new doctoral degree in behavioral health, has not yet been recognized for licensure in any state. By requiring that each student already has a license to practice the program ensures that upon graduation, students will have a doctoral degree from an accredited university and a master's license to practice integrated behavioral care. In addition, the supply of existing therapists far exceeds the demand for patients in traditional settings. By upgrading master's level providers to integrated care doctoral care providers we are shifting clinicians from the oversupply in traditional settings to meet the demand to treat patients who are currently *not* being treated in primary care. This is good for patients, the healthcare system, and DBH graduates.

The DBH program is provisionally accredited by the National Institute of Behavioral Health Quality (NIBHQ), an accreditation developed by the National Alliance of Professional Psychology Providers. The vision is that other universities or professional schools adopt the DBH as a new applied doctoral degree for behavioral providers in integrated care settings, and that the NIBHQ becomes the professional accreditation organization for these emerging programs. In addition to giving clinicians credit for their master's degree credits towards the DBH degree, the program also gives clinicians credit for between 1500 and 3000 hours of supervised internship experience that were part of their master's degree and master's license. The DBH is designed to build on existing competencies in psychotherapy with specific new competencies for a doctoral level behavioral care provider in an integrated care setting. The DBH internship hours (400) on top of the prior supervised internship hours are seen as sufficient for achieving proficiency, provided the student achieves the benchmarks based on assessment of competency in the program.

In addition, the DBH program curriculum and internship program is designed to largely meet current and emerging APA and ASPPB standards for both a doctoral psychology program and internship experience. This includes the APA Guidelines and Principles for Accreditation of Programs in Professional Psychology, the recommendations of the APA Task Force on the Assessment of Competence in Professional Psychology, and the ASPPB Guidelines on Internship Experience for Licensure. Admittedly, it may be a long and winding trajectory from establishment and credentialing of a new program to state licensure. Designing a program that largely meets existing state license board requirements for a doctoral degree license in behavioral care is prudent and logical.

## Career Opportunities for the DBH Behavioral Care Provider

The key career path for the DBH behavioral care provider is the primary care or related medical setting. However, a number of other career paths seem appropriate for the provision of integrated behavioral care:

- SAMHSA is awarding grants for pilot projects to locate primary care and nursing providers in traditional mental health and substance abuse treatment settings
- Health plans, carve-outs, and other vendors continue to offer disease management and case management programs using telephonic outreach to engage high-cost, high-risk patients with co-morbid medical and behavioral conditions
- Large employer groups are searching for solutions to address the high cost of lost productivity and disability due to behavioral conditions. The use of EAP services is on the rise and a potential career path.
- There is a proliferation of companies developing ehealth interventions for behavioral and medical conditions. Clinicians familiar with ehealth and integrat-

ed care are likely to contribute significantly to design and evaluation of such programs.

Finally, traditional education in behavioral health leaves clinicians with the perception that their only options are to accept a relatively low fee for service reimbursement from payers, or to opt out of insurance panels. The DBH program emphasis on behavioral entrepreneurship is designed to help clinicians think outside of the box for new business start-up opportunities.

## Summary and Next Steps

The Doctorate of Behavioral Health represents a model for radical reform in the education of doctoral level, behavioral care providers. The program is designed to meet the emerging needs of healthcare reform to produce clinicians who are able to provide clinical services in integrated care settings with the explicit goal of improved clinical outcome and demonstrating medical cost offset. The DBH curriculum and training progression are based on a cohesive, sequential program of study that will prepare graduates with the clinical, medical literacy, and entrepreneurial skills necessary to thrive in the 21st century healthcare system.

The DBH program has been very successful in terms of student enrollment, retention, and satisfaction. The online component of the program has been very successful and continues to evolve based on student and faculty recommendations. Internship placements have been successful as evidenced by both successful agreements with primary care and related sites across the country and high physician satisfaction with the role of the DBH in practice. The key focus over the first two years of the program development has been on quality. Developing the course content, identifying adjunct faculty, and especially developing online learning that is highly interactive complimented by on-site residency programs have been critical areas of development. The DBH program is now turning to a number of strategic initiatives designed to improve both the quality of training and education and the opportunities for our graduates in the workforce.

First, the program is focused on beginning to develop a research base for publication on areas such as clinical outcomes in primary care and the impact of behavioral interventions on workplace productivity. A formal physician survey is under development in order to measure pre- and post-satisfaction with the addition of a DBH to the physician practice. Our vision is to develop a comprehensive research base in order to publish DBH program performance metrics.

Second, the program will focus on initiatives designed to enhance collaboration between DBH clinicians and practicing psychologists. Many patients identified in primary care settings will require referral for specialty behavioral health services such as long-term psychotherapy, psychological and neuropsychological assessment, and other specialty services that are out of scope for the DBH practice. The DBH program will partner with psychologists nationwide who have expertise in integrated care and are interested in providing supervision to DBH students. The DBH program is also establishing a national network of psychologist-led integrated care programs to serve as internship sites for our students. Business partnerships between DBH clinicians and psychologists on projects such as screening and referral and population-based interventions are anticipated. It is also anticipated that the DBH program will offer certificate and CEU training programs to psychologists in order to offer many of the unique components of the program to current doctoral clinicians who are not interested in graduate coursework.

Third, the DBH program will take steps to substantially increase enrollment in order to move the program to a scale nationally and internationally. The program will move from enrollment only in the fall of each year to rolling enrollment with admissions in fall, spring, and summer semesters. National marketing programs will increase substantially. The program will move from targeting largely master's level licensed behavioral clinicians to enrolling master's level ancillary healthcare professionals such as nurses, dieticians, and occupational therapists. The DBH program has applied for trademark and efforts are now in motion to establish regional DBH programs via franchising at other universities across the United States.

Fourth, the program will move towards international student recruitment, clinician training and research collaboration. The same drivers that are pushing the United States healthcare market towards reform such as integrated and improved chronic disease management are operating internationally. As a pilot program, the DBH is preparing to offer continuing education on key components of the program to a community health center in Beijing, China. Recruitment of Chinese students will follow, and it is anticipated that research collaboration will be established between at least one major Chinese university and the DBH program. Pending the success of these programs similar opportunities are envisioned in other countries. These initiatives will also present career opportunities for DBH students and graduates.

The DBH program embraces the concept of "disruptive technology and business model change" outlined by Christensen et al. (2009). The DBH program has achieved dramatic success in a very short period and has achieved positive recognition nationally and now internationally. At its core, the program remains committed to the vision of Nicholas A. Cummings, who for over five decades has advocated for the creation of a new breed of doctoral behavioral clinicians who are equally adept at psychotherapy, integrated care, and entrepreneurship. The time is finally right for this program, as forces for reform both in clinical education and training and the healthcare marketplace have dovetailed to create a need for a radical new approach to training doctoral behavioral clinicians, to return them to prominence in terms of recognition and income. While the DBH program is still in its infancy, all signs point towards long-term success in radical transformation of our healthcare system.

# References

American Psychological Association (2006). *APA Task Force on the Assessment of Competence in Professional Psychology: Final Report.* Retrieved April 2, 2010 from http://www.apa.org/ed/resources/competency-revised.pdf

American Psychological Association Commission on Accreditation (2007). *Guidelines and principles for accreditation of programs in professional psychology.* Washington, DC: American Psychological Association.

Antos, J, Bertko, J et al (2009). Bending the curve: effective steps to address long-term healthcare spending growth. *American Journal of Managed Care,* 15:676-680.

Association of State and Provincial Psychology Boards (2009). *Guidelines on internship experience for licensure.* Retrieved April 2, 2010 from http://www.asppb.net/files/public/Final_Prac_Guidelines_1_31_09.pdf

Chaffee, O'Donohue, WT, and Cummings, NA (in preparation). A military integrated care project demonstration.

Cummings NA. (2002). Medical cost offset as a roadmap to behavioral entrepreneurship: lessons from the Hawaii project, (pps. 27-45). In Cummings NA, WT O'Donohue, KE Ferguson (Eds.). The impact of medical cost offset on practice and research: making it work for you. Reno, NV: Context Press.

Cummings, NA and O'Donohue, WT (2008). *Eleven blunders that cripple psychotherapy in America: A remedial unblundering.* New York: Routledge.

Cummings NA, Cummings JL (2000). *The essence of psychotherapy: reinventing the art for the new era of data.* San Diego, CA: Harcourt Press.

Cummings NA, Cummings JL. (2005). Behavioral interventions for somatizers within the primary care setting (pps. 49-70). In Cummings NA, O'Donohue WT, Naylor EV (Eds.). *Psychological Approaches to Chronic Disease Management.* Reno, NV: Context Press.

Cummings NA, Sayama, M (1995). *Focused psychotherapy: a casebook of brief intermittent psychotherapy throughout the life cycle.* Madison, CT: Psychological Press.

DeMers, ST, Van Horen, BA, Rodolfa, ER (2008). Changes in training and practice of psychologists: Current challenges for licensing boards. *Professional Psychology: Practice and Research, 39,* 473-79.

France, CR, Belar, CD, et al (2008). Application of the competency model to clinical health psychology. *Professional Psychology: Research and Practice, 39,* 573-80.

Frank, RG, Goldman, HH, McGuire, TG (2009). Trends in mental health cost growth: An expanded role for management? *Health Affairs, 28,* 649-59.

Fries J, Koop C, Beadle C. Reducing healthcare costs by reducing the need and demand for medical services. *New England J of Medicine.* 1993; 329:321-25.

Harmon SC, Lambert MJ, Smart DM, et al. (2007). Enhancing outcome for potential treatment failures: therapist-client feedback and clinical support tools. *Psychotherapy Research, 17,* 379-92.

Hu XH, Bull SA, Hunkeler EM, et al. (2004). Incidence and duration of side effects and those rated as bothersome with selective serotonin reuptake inhibitor treatment for depression: patient report versus physician estimate. J Clin Psychiatry. 2004; 65:959-65.

James, L, and O'Donohue, WT (2008). *The primary care toolkit: Practical resources for the integrated behavioral care provider.* New York: Springer.

Kathol RG, McAlpine D, Kishi Y, et al. (2005). General medical and pharmacy claims expenditures in users of behavioral health services. *Journal of General Internal Medicine.* 2005; 20:160-67.

Katon W, Lin E, Von Korff M, Russo J, Lipscomb P, Bush T. Somatization: a spectrum of severity. *American Journal of Psychiatry.* 1991; 148:34-40

Kay-Lambkin FJ, Baker AL, Lewin TJ, & Carr VJ (2009). Computer-based psychological treatment for comorbid depression and problematic alcohol and/or cannabis use: a randomized controlled trial of clinical efficacy. *Addiction, 104*:378-88.

Kessler, R.C., Barber, C., Beck, A., Berglund, P., Cleary, P.D., McKenas, D., Pronk, N., Simon, G., Stang, P., Üstün, T.U., Wang, P. (2003). The World Health Organization Health and Work Performance Questionnaire (HPQ). *Journal of Occupational and Environmental Medicine, 45,* 156-174.

Knaevelsrud C & Maercker A (2007). Internet-based treatment for PTSD reduces distress and facilitates the development of a strong therapeutic alliance: A randomized controlled clinical trial. *BMC Psychiatry. 19*:7-13.

Loeppke R, Taitel M, Richling D, et al. (2007). Health and productivity as a business strategy. *Journal of Occupational and Environmental Medicine.* 49:712-21.

Mackinnon A, Griffiths KM, & Christensen H. (2008). Comparative randomised trial of online cognitive-behavioural therapy and an information website for depression: 12-month outcomes. *British Journal of Psychiatry 192*(2):130-4.

Marks, I & Cavanagh, K (2009). Computer-aided psychological treatments: evolving issues. *Annual Rev Clin Psychol,5:*121-41

McDaniel, SH, Schroeder, C, Belar, CD, Hargrove, DS, Freeman, EL (2002). A training curriculum for professional psychologists in primary care. *Professional Psychology: Research and Practice, 33*, 65-72.

Miller SD, Duncan BL, Brown J, Sorrell R, Chalk MB (2006). Using formal client feedback to improve retention and outcome: making ongoing, real-time assessment feasible. *Journal of Brief Therapy, 5*, 5-22.

O'Donohue, WT, and Boland (in preparation). The Rube Goldberg model of clinical training: Toward the explication of core competencies.

O'Donohue, WT, Byrd, MR, Cummings, NA, Henderson, DA (2005). *Behavioral integrative care: Treatments that work in the primary care setting.* New York: Brunner-Routledge.

O'Donohue, WT, and Buchanan, JA (2003). The mismeasure of psychologists: A review of the psychometrics of licensing requirements. In O'Donohue, WT and Ferguson, K (Eds.), *The handbook of professional ethics for psychologists.* Thousand Oaks, CA: Sage Publications.

O'Donohue, WT, Cummings, NA, Cummings, JL (2008). The unmet educational agenda in integrated care. *Journal of Clinical Psychology in Medical Settings. 28*, 94-100.

O'Donohue, WT, Laygo, R, and Cummings, N (2001). Hawaii integrated healthcare demonstration project. Reno, NV: The Cummings Foundation for Behavioral Health.

Olfson, M, Marcus, SC (2009). National patterns of antidepressant medication treatment. *Archives of General Psychiatry, 66*, 848-56.

Prochaska, JO, Redding CA, Evers KE (2008). The transtheoretical model of behavior change. In Glanz, K., Lewis, F.M., & Rimer, B.K. (Eds.), *Health behavior and health education: theory, research and practice (3rd ed.)*, (pp. 97-121). San Francisco: Jossey-Bass.

Reger MA & Gahm GA (2009). A meta-analysis of the effects of internet and computer-based cognitive-behavioral treatments for anxiety. *J Clin Psychol, 65*:53-75.

Robinson, P and Reiter, J (2007). *Behavioral consultation and primary care: A guide to integration*. New York: Springer.

Simon, GE (2002). Evidence review: efficacy and effectiveness of antidepressant treatment in primary care. General Hospital Psychiatry. 24:213-24.

Satterfield, JM (2003). Core competencies of the primary care provider in an integrated team. In Cummings, NA, O'Donohue, WT, and Ferguson, KE (Eds.). *Behavioral health as primary care: Beyond efficacy to effectiveness.* Reno, NV: Context Press.

Smith GR, Monson RA, Ray DC. (1986). Patients with multiple unexplained symptoms: their characteristics, functional health, and healthcare utilization. *Archives of Internal Medicine.* 146:69-72.

Strosahl, K (2005). Training behavioral health and primary care providers for integrated care: A core competencies approach. In O'Donohue, WT, Byrd, MR, Cummings, NA and Henderson, DA (Eds.). *Behavioral integrative care: Treatments that work in the primary care setting*. New York: Brunner-Routledge.

Van Schaik, DJ, Klijn, AF, van Hout, HP, et al. (2004). Patients' preferences in the treatment of depression in primary care. Gen Hospital Psychiatry. 26:184-89.

Chapter 8

# Health and Behavior: Expanding the Role of Psychologists in Skilled Nursing Facilities

*Presented at the Conference on Restoring Psychotherapy as the First-Line Intervention in Behavioral Health and reprinted by permission.*

*Joseph M. Casciani, PhD*

would like first, to thank the organizers of this conference and Dr. Cummings for inviting me to speak on a subject that is near and dear to my heart, namely, expanding the role of psychologists in long term care settings. I have spent much of my professional career not only working in the field of geropsychology, but also training others and helping to prepare them to provide psychological services to the older adult population. In my talk, I am going to give you my perspective on how and why psychologists can be central to patient care in nursing facilities, help patients improve when possible and to help them better cope when improvement is not possible.

To begin, I will give some background on nursing homes in the U.S., including the incidence of medical and psychiatric diagnoses, especially depression. Then, we will briefly review traditional psychological services with this population. And, in the third and final section, I will address the trends and opportunities that are presented to us, based on what I see as the major shifts in patient needs and how we as psychologists and mental health professionals can meet these needs.

Behavioral health services are becoming a growing force to be reckoned with in the health care system in our country. The authors of this statement maintain that the greatest payoff in reducing morbidity and mortality will come from improving the delivery of behavioral health services in primary care. And for today's presentation, I would like to ask that you change the phrase "primary care" to "long term care" and follow me along as I make my case. So, this sentence changes to: "A review of the evidence shows that many forms of behavioral health services, particularly when delivered as part of **long term care**, can be central to such an improvement (Blount et al., 2007).

## Part 1. Overview of Nursing Homes

There are approximately 1.43 million residents in skilled nursing facilities (SNF) in the U.S. (Hyer, 2009). The number of homes has been steady, or declining slightly, and now number around 16,000. The census in most homes is below capacity, and the occupancy rate is around 86%. But, the length of stay is changing: approximately 20% are in and out of the facility in less than three months. I maintain that number would be higher if behavioral health services were more readily available. I will cover this in more detail later. Long term stay then is about 80% of the admissions, and long term stay is defined as more than eight weeks. It is important to note that these numbers are definitely shifting. The number of patients who are staying less than three months in a SNF has doubled in the last few years. Interestingly, the percentage of patients staying long term has not changed. And, just for additional facts, most admissions come from acute care hospitals, about a fourth come from those living at home, and the remainders are admitted from assisted living facilities and other SNFs.

A breakdown of admitting diagnoses, presents no real surprises as to the need for around-the-clock nursing care. What struck me when I first saw that 16.6% of nursing home residents have mental disorders, while 14.5% have actual mental illnesses, was how underlying psychological factors must also be part of the remainder composed of medical conditions. Twenty-three percent of the patients have diseases of the circulatory system—are there emotional factors present, and have hypertension and poor stress management been part of the clinical picture and lifestyle of the patient? For mental disorders, that is obvious as far as a history of psychiatric illness is concerned. Another category, diseases of the nervous system, encompasses stroke, dementias, and related cognitive disorders that have a strong psychological component as to adjustment to and management of the disease. Even miscellaneous injury and fractures, like a fall and hip fracture, raise questions as to how does a patient's outlook toward the future impact his or her recovery and potential to return home. Diseases of the respiratory system, like asthma and emphysema, is another category that has many co-morbid psychological issues, including anxiety, demanding and helpless behavior patterns, and a tendency to panic when breathing becomes more labored. In any discussion of the underlying complications to these medical conditions, we find that the term "co-morbid" is a very apt way to describe the interface between psychological and medical. A co-morbid factor intensifies or complicates management of or recovery from the primary condition.

A decided trend has occurred over the years in nursing homes. As we look at behavioral problems in the long-term care facility, I've always found it helpful to differentiate between two models of care. One is the traditional model of custodial care. When looking at the negative stereotype of the nursing home, the custodial model represents much of what was undesirable about these settings, and is much less common today than even a decade ago. The custodial care model provided for the basic needs of patients, their food, cleanliness, medication, and whatever medical care was necessary. But, there were no expectations for keeping the patient at his or her highest level of functioning, nor was there an emphasis on individualizing the psychosocial care. Fortunately, that traditional model has evolved into what we call a contemporary functional capacities model. This was the paradigm shift that took place in the 1980s, the decade of nursing home reform. OBRA, the Omnibus Budget Reconciliation Act of 1986, for the first time, addressed nursing home patients' rights, including a freedom from unnecessary physical and chemical restraints, and a greater emphasis on psychosocial needs. Then, only a few years later, Congress mandated that psychologists should be authorized providers for the Medicare system. One of the very positive effects of this shift in caregiving models is that we are now really interested in looking at different areas of functioning of the residents and developing individually-tailored care plans, based on their different levels of functioning. For example, we need to consider what the behavior capacities are, what the communication skills are, the social behaviors, the physical condition, psychological condition, capacity for self-care and activities of daily living (ADLs), and cognitive functioning. Each of these major domains plays a role in planning the most appropriate level of treatment for the individual, based on the mix of strengths and weaknesses. We really must make the most of what the residual capacities are of the individual resident, and incorporate these in the treatment plan. Of course, this new model also gives the behavioral health professional the weight or the authority to help with the comprehensive assessment and identify residual or remaining strengths of the patient.

To get back to the nursing home overview, OBRA gives you an idea of the caregiving problems and demands presented by the patients. Most have serious problems with activities of daily living, and the majority have problems with continence and bowel or bladder control. As for the staffing requirements, because these facilities are "skilled nursing," a licensed nurse is on staff twenty-four hours, seven days a week. And, just as a note, 90% of facilities are understaffed, which should not be a surprise to anyone. But, consider the demands, responsibilities, and working conditions in many buildings, and we can easily see the reason for the understaffing. But, this is the subject of another talk.

Of the incidence of co-exiting psychiatric diagnoses in the nursing home population, 46.5% manifest dementia, while an overlapping 46.8% reveal depression. Rarely, however, are these diagnoses the primary reason for admission, but either as a formal DSM diagnosis or a manifestation of these clinical signs, we can easily recognize that psychiatric symptomatology is prevalent in these settings.

The OBRA in-depth investigations of depression in older adults, and verified by the National Institute of Health, painted the perfect picture for mental health needs in nursing homes. The investigation concluded that the highest incidence of depression in late life is in nursing homes, there is an unmet need for psychological treatment, and anti-depressant medications may help, but **psychological treatment is always needed.** And the best, most salient point that this report reinforced is that depression in older adults is never normal. It may be common, highly characteristic of this age group, but it should never be considered normal. The "ageist" attitudes, like "She's 90 years old—wouldn't you be depressed?" are finally dying off, fortunately. Though we do still hear a comment like, "He's got multiple medical problems, is in failing health—what's a psychologist going to do for him?"

When depression is left untreated, anywhere, but certainly in nursing homes, there are consequences. First, depression is treatable. It may be accompanying a serious medical diagnosis like congestive heart failure. But, depression should be considered an excess disability, just like hearing loss in a patient with advanced dementia. We should treat what we can, even though the patient can't be cured of all debilities. Depression leaves a person more dependent on caregivers, lacking a "self-care" mindset, and more likely to somaticize his or her problems, which increases the demand on medical care and services. Lastly, depression makes a person more vulnerable to suicide and a reduced quality of life.

We've all seen mnemonics for remembering lists of symptoms. This is a good one, from the National Initiative for the Care of the Elderly (NICE) in Toronto, Canada: www.nicenet.ca :

SIG E CAPS:

Sleep is disturbed
Interest is decreased
Guilt feelings
Energy is less than usual

Concentration is poor
Appetite is disturbed
Psychomotor agitation or agitation
Suicidal ideation

And here is a nice array of depression screening tools, some of which are in public domain and some of which are copyrighted by the test publishers:

- Geriatric Depression Scale
- Cornell Scale for Depression in Dementia
- Beck Depression Scale

- Depression Status Inventory
- Brief Symptom Inventory (53 or 18 item versions)
- Hospital Anxiety and Depression Scale
- Patient Health Questionnaire 2-Stage Screening Scale (PHQ and PHQ-9)
- Center for Epidemiological Studies-Depression Scale
- Hamilton Rating Scale for Depression

# Part 2. Traditional Psychological Services

In this second section, I'd like to offer some insights into our role as psychologists with the nursing home population.

One of the best resources I found for this work was a book written by Dr. Bob Knight a few decades ago, *Psychotherapy with Older Adults*. He discusses the adjustments we must make as psychotherapists with the aged. Of course, we now are well aware of these issues, like the constant interplay between physical and the psychological—the attitudes, worries, and self-talk, about the losses and physical decline that accompanies the aging process. The increased introspection and interiority common in this age group make the psychotherapy process often a welcome respite from nurses, needles, dressings, and pills. We must also recognize that defenses can be very fragile in older adults; denial may be the only means or tool a person has to manage some very distressing and unpleasant realities. We have to respect this coping mechanism that is barely effective and rather primitive. When you tell your patient who is pressing to go home, "You're not ever going home again because your two daughters sold your house and are now tangled up in a legal dispute over your estate, and there's no money left to pay for your medical care," that's probably a contraindicated psychological strategy. There is a place for reality orientation, but this isn't one of them.

One other important point about psychotherapy with older adults is the need for education about the benefits and the process of therapy. We don't disguise our profession, but we should be ready to take the spotlight off "psychological problems." Older adults are still uncomfortable admitting to feeling depressed, or having "personal problems." I would always introduce myself as "Dr. Casciani, a psychologist, and I'd like to see how you are getting along and what we can do to better help you." One good way to build an alliance and tap their views about placement is to ask a question like, "What's your doctor told you about your need to be here?" We all know what the answer to this question. I always feel like Johnny Carson's character, Karnack, The Magician, who knows the answer before the question is raised.

There are some fundamental themes in psychological treatment with nursing home patients. Themes like empowerment, in the face of increased dependency and helplessness, a loss of joy and pleasure in life, and a steady succession of failures and losses not only are grist for the therapeutic mill, but are very real issues about the transition from living to dying. Robert Butler's, one of our country's great gerontologists, used the life review process to help older adults view successes and triumphs that they experienced in the past as a way to help employ some of the same determination and resilience as they face new challenges in their later years. The A-R-K mnemonic helps us to remember basic approaches for the depressed: attention, reassurance—though not false reassurance—and kind firmness (i.e., gentle pushes toward recovery or toward new behavior). And, I've always found a solution-oriented approach to be very effective with these patients. We don't need to know why—I'm of the mind that insight alone doesn't do much to change behavior—we need to look at engaging in new behaviors that are getting us closer toward the goal. When you ask a patient, "How will you know you're not depressed anymore?" and she says, "I'd get out of bed and open the drapes to let the sun in," that becomes the new behavioral prescription for this patient. One other point about psychotherapy with this older age group is that the patient himself sets the goals for treatment. Any change has to be inner directed, or they won't last.

We know more today about suicide risk in nursing homes. Some of the risk factors, and some of the best predictors of self-harm behaviors. Risk factors include first of all physical illness. Other risk factors are chronic, severe pain, debilitating disease or terminal illness, depression, Alzheimer's disease, and a history of alcohol or substance abuse. Predictors for suicide include undesirable transfer, a new medical condition, recent medication change, an increase in medication non-compliance, and an expression of hopelessness. (Two points to consider with suicide risk in older adults: first, the attempt-to-success ratio is much higher than it is for middle-aged and younger adults: 2:1 vs. 7:1; and, there are many high risk, sub-intentional behaviors like refusing medication, reckless physical maneuvers like climbing out of bed to a wheelchair or Geri-chair, or reduced food intake.

There are two broad treatment approaches. There is the group of patients with functional disorders, depression, generalized anxiety disorder, adjustment disorder. In these cases, we apply a therapeutic treatment, that is psychotherapy, and generally, the condition improves and the signs and symptoms do not return. The second group is comprised of organic disorders—these are unchangeable conditions, where the symptoms are irreversible and the treatment is permanently required. This is where we get the term "prosthetic environment," just like any prosthesis is permanently required. We do not expect the leg to grow back after the prosthesis has been applied for six months. Rather, the environment itself must be arranged to make up for or replace what is missing because of the dementia or cognitive impairment. Communication, cues and directions, explanations, and all caregiving approaches must provide the extraordinary level of detail and patience required by patients who are cognitively impaired.

When we discuss the topic of dementia, we have to remember that it is a syndrome or a collection or cluster of symptoms, marked chiefly by diffuse intellectual deterioration. This intellectual deterioration is accompanied by behavior problems and emotional changes or emotional deregulation. The term dementia itself does not say anything about the cause or whether it is reversible or not. That is because there are irreversible types of dementia and reversible types of dementia. Some of the causes of irreversible dementia include degenerative diseases such as Alzheimer's disease, vascular dementia, which is a series of mini strokes that affect the cognitive functioning and result in deterioration over time. There is traumatic dementia, infectious dementias, toxic dementias, all of these are considered irreversible and primary. That is why we use the term primary degenerative dementia as another name for Alzheimer's disease. Some secondary causes of dementia, which is the reversible type, may include psychiatric conditions such as depression, and nutritional or dietary deficiencies, and certain medications can also produce some changes in functioning that resemble or mimic dementia. It should be stated, though, that in long term care settings, most of the dementias that we see, probably 90% or more of the dementia cases, are of the irreversible type.

As we discuss difficult behaviors and understanding what the syndrome of dementia is all about, it is helpful to categorize the triggers or the causes of these difficult behaviors. The first category is made up of **physical and emotional** causes. Obviously, the cognitive changes that come with dementia will contribute to a lot of difficult behaviors, but also sensory losses such as vision and hearing, acute and chronic illness, psychological conditions such as depression or anxiety, medical conditions such as UTI, bladder infection, constipation, and fatigue. Any of these physical and emotional causes constitutes one group of the causes of difficult behavior. A second category includes **environmental causes.** Too much stimulation or too little stimulation, a lack of structure, unfamiliar people, unfamiliar places, changes that the patient does not understand or no one has communicated, are the environmental causes that will contribute to significantly difficult behaviors. A third category has to do with the task at hand. If it is too complicated, if there are too many steps, if it's something that creates too much of a demand on the individual, that will often result in a physical or emotional outburst. Lastly, communicational difficulties will contribute to a lot of these behavior problems. Any type of aphasia, the inability to communicate one's own needs or ideas or wants, creates a lot of frustration and more vulnerability to behavioral problems.

It is important to distinguish depression from dementia. As mentioned, depression can sometimes mimic dementia. It can produce some of the cognitive changes that we see often with dementia, sometimes referred to as pseudodementia, or false dementia. Some of the unique differences between these two conditions are that with depression, it tends to be a more sudden onset. Dementia has a more gradual, slow, insidious onset. In depression, we often have early morning awakening. Whereas in dementia, we don't have that difficulty with sleep. With depression, there is often a history of psychiatric problems whereas that is usually absent in dementia. The major change or distinction that I have always witnessed with depression vs. dementia, is that in the depressed person there is an emphasis or a highlighting of any losses particularly memory problems or concentration difficulties. In contrast, in the dementia patient we get that covered up, or masked, or denied. The person does not admit to having these difficulties. They really want to hide the cognitive changes that are taking place. There is also a pattern of memory difficulty with depression, but it's not consistent. It tends to be manifested as difficulty with recent and remote events whereas with dementia it tends to be recent or short-term memory problems. Sundowning is a characteristic that we see in dementia patients and that occurs toward the end of the day and it is linked to the sunset, largely due to the loss of structure and changes in schedule; the dementia person has more difficulty with this loss of structure whereas we do not see it so much with the depressed person.

The following principles are what I consider to be the most important aspects of managing problem behaviors in the nursing home.

1. The first has to do with a calm and reassuring environment. We need to be sure it's not over stimulating. We cannot have too much going on in the environment, too much stimulation, such as the television, radio, and overhead PA system. Any of these excessive stimuli create anxiety and restlessness in the individual because the dementia patient, as we know, has difficulty processing complex information, and has difficulty tuning out and filtering unwanted or unnecessary sounds. So, with excessive stimulation we create the setting, the opportunity, and the risk for rising agitation and the potential for behavior problems. The more secure and more safe the individual feels, the less anxiety he experiences, and the less anxiety, the less chance of behavioral outburst.

2. Maintain consistency in all routines whenever possible. That means familiar caregivers, familiar rooms for activities, and seating arrangements in the dining room, roommates, and anything that is being provided for this individual should be the same, and as predictable and consistent as possible.

3. Keep expectations realistic. As was said earlier, the dementia person tends to deny, disguise, or mask the extent of cognitive changes that are occurring internally. As a result, it is very easy to overestimate what the person is understanding or comprehending in our communications. So we might think the person is perfectly okay with the explanation that we are giving, but in fact, it likely is way too complicated for her to process. Even though she

acts as though she is understanding and following what we are saying, the result is a lot of frustration on the caregiver's part and the patient's part because of that inability to fully understand and follow that communication.

4. Provide opportunities for success. Help the patient to continue doing whatever self-care is possible and avoid any unnecessary feelings of loss and failure. Tap into those residual strengths, reinforce them, have the person continue whatever he or she is able to continue. Give him that opportunity to feel good about himself, to have some sense of positive self-esteem in the face of all of the other losses that are taking place.

5. Keep communication and language as simple as possible, limited to short phrases and directions. If the patient cannot follow the communication, that is a frequent source of behavioral outbursts. When repeating statements or questions, repeat yourself exactly to avoid confusion that comes with delayed comprehension.

6. Use distraction when dealing with the argumentative or combative patient; distract him onto another topic or a different point of discussion. When the patient is demanding to go home, for example, rather than try and debate with the person, it is usually preferable to shift the focus of the conversation. With this patient who is demanding to go home, engage him in a conversation for a few minutes about his home. What was home like, who was at home, who did he live with, where did he grow up, what was it like in his family growing up? Shifting to this more desirable, pleasing conversation avoids the power struggle that we are not going to win with the dementia-afflicted person. Logic and reasoning can be very ineffective with patients who have any type of cognitive impairment.

7.  As a general principal, we want to use isolation when the patient becomes agitated and move him to another room or another that is less stressful and less stimulating. When settled down again, the person can return back to the activity.

8.  Provide the extraordinary structure and cues for the individual to make up for what is missing. This is sometimes referred to as reality orientation, but it must take place around the clock. We must communicate what is happening to the individual. Explain what is going to happen. Explain what just happened, what the daily schedule is, what the day and date and seasons and holidays are. We see the activity boards in the nursing home. These are there for a reason, to provide that extraordinary structure, although sometimes they can be too complicated and they tend to be more a source of confusion than providing any reassurance and external cues. Whatever structure, communication, and reality orientation we can provide, the better. In the absence of this, the person gets more anxious. The more the anxiety level goes up, the more likely he is to engage in some type of problem behaviors.

9.  It is always important to remind caregivers to not take these behavioral outbursts personally. Often, these difficulties have very little to do with what we are providing as caregivers. The patient is reacting to a lot of triggers, internal triggers, and external triggers, things that are going on inside and outside. The fact that we are there doesn't mean that we are contributing to that. Although inadvertently we may be, we still must understand how and why those actions are taking place so we do not get caught up in them emotionally, and so we do not react in a defensive way. We should refrain from expressing

our judgment or opinion or disdain for these behaviors. These are, in a vast majority of cases, unintentional behaviors that the person has no control over or very little control over as a result of the dementing condition.

# Part 3. Trends and Opportunities

It is important to discuss the shift in the nursing home admission patterns and the change in population, and what this means for psychologists. A study published by the National Hospital Discharge Survey (NHDS), 2004, gives a picture of nursing home admissions, divided into the "short stayers" and the "long stayers". Short stay is defined as up to eight weeks; "long stayers" are generally over eight weeks, and on average, up to two years. "Short stayers" are considered sub-acute, or post-acute, with a variety of issues, usually very short-term rehab issues. These short term admissions will receive intensive treatments, and return to the community whenever possible. The "long stayers" are those that don't succeed in their rehab (if that was the plan), or they are known at the outset that long term placement will be necessary. Often, there may be other more serious medical conditions with the long term, chronic care population, such as cognitive impairment or a combination of cognitive and physical debility.

Many skilled nursing facilities are converting even more long term care beds to the Part A beds, technically defined as Medicare Part A. Medicare will pay for that portion of the nursing home stay, as long as the patient is eligible to receive these benefits. Once the patient gets off Part A, no longer qualifies for Part A, or loses Part A eligibility, the patient either returns home or more likely is transferred to a long-term care unit in the facility. The "short stayers", then, by definition, are the Part A patients, and Medicare reimburses the facility for Part A stays. After Part A lapses, the patient's stay is covered by out-of-pocket costs until the person qualifies for Medicaid, and in some instances by special insurance policies covering long term care.

The National Hospital Discharge Survey also reflected a trend that the admissions from hospitals and "quicker and sicker." The length of stay is shorter in the acute care hospitals. There are more transfers from the acute to the sub-acute and there's a greater flow of patients through the system. And, of course, there is a higher acuity, but these patients end up in long-term care nonetheless. This means that we are seeing more admissions, and more discharge activity. The recommendations from the NHDS report were strongly advocating greater interdisciplinary collaboration, including different types of staff expertise and staff input. And, again, the behavioral health professional is central to this collaboration, with an emphasis on interdisciplinary involvement, discussion, and participation in treatment planning with other team members.

### *Treatment with Short Term and Long Term Patients*

Short term treatment usually involves patients with hip fracture, stroke, amputations, knee surgery, generally whatever can be treated in up to three months. Medicare will pay for 100 days, or roughly three months of sub-acute care. So what are we trying to understand as a behavioral health consultant, and contribute to the team? Can we help the staff understand what this person's functioning is in some important areas so they can more effectively work with their patients? For example, what is the cognitive status, since dementia can easily mask the extent of comprehension and recognition about the rehab process? What can the patient really understand? Can they follow instructions?

Is there any underlying or pre-existing emotional disorder, or mental disorder? How much will that interfere with the person's participation in rehab? Or, is there a personality disorder or some characterological disturbance that is going to impact the patient's compliance, participation, or engagement in his rehab program? If there is depression, what does it look like? Is it a reactive depression? Is it major depression? Does it impact this person's future outlook? Does it create a barrier for the patient to become involved? Is the patient saying, "Well, what's the use? I'm not going to be normal again. My future is very bleak and negative. I don't think I'm going to get involved?" So, as we are able to identify these underlying barriers, of course, we can offer the approach and offer some treatment and help staff understand how to optimize their caregiving approach. Similarly, with anxiety, pain, or whatever symptoms this individual is experiencing, as we can identify it, communicate it, and help care plan it with the rest of the staff, the patient is more likely to get more comprehensive, effective treatment program.

The "long stayers", in contrast, are the patients that are placed for more than eight weeks. These are the patients that have not rehabilitated successfully and consequently are likely to remain in long term placement. However, it is important to point out that they can be re-referred for rehab if they become eligible later on. If we are working with some of these "long stayers" and we see that the person's depression is lifting and the motivation is more favorable, we can make a recommendation that this patient be reconsidered for another series of rehab treatment. This is a common occurrence. But without that involvement, without our input, and without our observation of these long stay patients, they may be relegated to long term placement.

What are the reasons for the longer stays? Some admitting diagnoses include Alzheimer's disease, all different types of dementia, as well as chronic lung disease, where the patient's respiratory distress is so great the patient requires daily nursing care. Additionally, strokes that have left the affected patient so debilitated that he cannot participate in his usual self-care activities require extra care and assistance in a nursing home. The cardiac conditions, such as congestive heart failure, and other deteriorative disease processes contribute to long term placement. Also in this category are problems with falls, where the presence of re-peated falls render this person unable to live independently. But, with proper fall management approaches and an appropriate level of motivation and reduced depression, these patients may be able to function at a higher level of functioning.

What does the mental health professional do with these primary medical conditions? With both the short and the long term admissions, the mental health consultant is generally helping the patient understand the emotional impact of the condition that led to his or her admission. She may have had a fall, but what are the accompanying emotional considerations here that this person needs help with? Secondly, we assess the values and perceptions of the patient regarding his future. What is this person's outlook like? Third, identify what kinds of barriers there are in partici-pating and benefiting from rehab treatment and help to overcome these barriers, working and collaborating closely with the rehab team. And fourth, offer therapeutic interventions that facilitate the safe and effective progress of rehab, effectively, helping the pa-tient to stay engaged once he does become involved in his physi-cal therapy. This means continually integrating the different ap-proaches among the team members, to ensure these patients are involved in and maximize their benefit from their treatment.

### *Interdisciplinary Collaboration*

As mental health professionals begin to do more work with nursing homes, we are seeing a trend towards patients being admitted with more acute illnesses, shorter stays after admission from the acute care hospital, and requiring more interdisciplin-ary care. These patients are not typically admitted for long term placement. On the contrary, they are being treated for acute con-ditions, such as a hip fracture or a stroke, (though they may have co-existing, chronic conditions), and are expected to return to in-dependent living when they progress through their short term rehabilitation. In order for mental health professionals to work with these patients, we must consider what the interactions are between the medical and psychological dimensions.

This brings the focus back to interdisciplinary collaboration, reiterating the major premise that the mind cannot separate from the body. The more we can advocate this interdisciplinary collaboration, the more we are accepted as a vital member of the team. This has been referred to as finding the seat at the table. As the saying goes, "If you don't have a seat at the table, you're on the menu." This is a familiar maxim used in politics and lobbying circles, but also is applicable to the presence of mental health professionals on the health care team. There is a need to "elbow" our way in to these interdisciplinary teams and represent what we can do with these patients, while supporting and facilitating this culture of integrated care. We must keep reiterating the premise that patients are not isolated from their disease, while emphasizing the importance of the behavioral health approaches in understanding, assessing and treating the patient, especially where the coping resources are limited or taxed.

One other point to be stressed while establishing our "seat at this table" is that our treatment approaches are characterized by brief, problem-focused interventions. It is not uncommon to hear nursing directors, social services personnel, and attending physicians question psychologists and LCSWs seeing their patients for months or years, yet nobody knows what the practitioner is working on, purportedly because this treatment has traditionally been deemed confidential and private by the practitioner. Of course, we must respect the confidentiality of our patients, but the interdisciplinary communication can occur without revealing confidential details or personal disclosures, because of the important focus on behavioral objectives and treatment goals, and patient motivations toward reaching these goals. Traditional, long term psychotherapy does not work well in this interdisciplinary setting, where the emphasis must be on shared understanding of treatment goals and barriers. In addition to stressing the short-term approach, we also must communicate in ways that the medical team understands. The team members want answers to quickly diagnose and fix problems. They need concise information and they need updates. So, this becomes part of our changing role as we become part of this interdisciplinary team.

Quote on American health care: *The design flaw is in the fact that the system operates as if biomedical and psychosocial were separate and parallel domains.* We would be hard pressed to find a more succinct statement about the absence of a behavioral health approach with the medical population that is filling all of our nursing home beds.

### *Introduction to Health and Behavior Codes*

A series of CPT codes authorized by Medicare in 2002 for psychologists, that, in my opinion, will ultimately do more to foster integration with primary care than any other development in the history of our profession.

In order to correctly use these codes, there are conditions that must be met. First, you can only use these with a medical diagnosis. You cannot use a DSM or psychiatric diagnosis with these codes. The second condition is that the physical disorder is always present and there are psychological factors that are influencing the course of the physical health problem. And thirdly, the patient's mental status must be at a suitable level for these interventions.

These procedures, therefore, allow the mental health professional to identify and address the factors that affect a person's physical functioning. For example, one would look at using H&B codes to affect a person's engaging in health risk behaviors, like poor diet and smoking. We can use these codes to address negative attitudes toward recovery. A major use of these codes is to focus on non-compliance with a medical treatment. These procedure codes are designed to help families understand what's going on with these patients, and how the families can be a part of the improvement. The H&B codes are also designed to help patients cope, or learn to better cope with the symptoms of the illness or learn to better manage the symptoms of the illness.

Although there is overlap between traditional psychotherapy and the H&B process, there are several distinguishing features. Are we not doing psychotherapy with these medical patients? Why is this H&B intervention any different from what we've always done? The chart below helps to point out these differences, on four dimensions (Casciani, 2004):

|  | **Psychotherapy** | **H&B** |
|---|---|---|
| **Diagnosis** | Mental illness and behavior disturbances | Physical illness or injury |
| **Primary Focus** | Affective relief, insight, decision making, resolve emotional condition | Psych factors that affect or interfere with physical functioning or recovery |
| **Goal** | Alleviate emotional disturbance, change behavior, growth | Improve health and well being |
| **Collaboration** | Emphasis on privacy and confidentiality | Encourages collaboration and co-treatment with primary care team |

On the first dimension, **diagnosis**, we are looking at mental illness and behavior disturbances in traditional psychotherapy, and a psychiatric diagnosis is required to bill for psychotherapy services. For H&B services, you can only use a physical illness, that is, the ICD-9

The **primary focus** of psychotherapy would be considered affective relief, insight, decision-making, and generally, help to resolve the emotional condition. The focus of H&B, in contrast, is on the psychological factors that affect or interfere with the physical functioning and recovery. The distinction may be subtle, but it is significant—focusing on the psychological factors that are impacting the physical. And, the **goal** with psychotherapy would generally be considered to be alleviating emotional distress, or behavior change, or growth. The goal with H&B is to improve health and well-being, including better management of or coping with the co-existing medical condition.

On the final dimension, we see a major distinction: the traditional psychotherapy model does not typically encourage **collaboration** with other caregivers or members of an interdisciplinary team, in view of the emphasis on privacy and confidentiality. But, by the very nature of the patient population with whom we are working, H&B requires collaboration, or co-treatment among the primary care team. This does not mean that the practitioner is disclosing intimate details. But, it does mean we are disclosing treatment goals, along with concrete, behavioral objectives. There can be an interdisciplinary discussion about interventions and treatment approaches. We are also disclosing patient's resistance or readiness for change. And, based on our knowledge of the patient's strengths and weaknesses, and optimum caregiving approaches and resistances, the mental health consultant can offer insights and recommendations to other team members.

We must always bear in mind the basic principles of behavior medicine: assessment focus is on rapid problem identification and limited problem definition; interventions focus on functional impairment, we must look and quantify outcomes, the work is open and collaborative, and we must have a tool box of assessment measures, interventions, and educational information.

### *H&B Assessment*

Health and behavior "assessment" procedures are used to identify the psychological, behavioral, emotional, cognitive and social factors important to the prevention, treatment or management of physical health problems. The focus of the assessment is not on mental health, but on the biopsychosocial factors important to physical health problems and treatments. In other words, the assessment codes are designed to identify co-morbid or underlying psychological factors that interfere with the recovery from or management of medical diagnoses, or conditions. That is, the assessment codes are used to identify underlying psychological, behavioral, emotional, cognitive, or social issues that interfere with or are impacted by a medical condition.

We are not administering a personality test or a projective test because we are not doing testing to diagnose a mental disorder. Instead, we're looking to identify what the level of anxiety or depression might be, how much stress is there, whether it is chronic or acute, what kind of dysfunctional attitudes or thinking are present. We need to identify the readiness for change: is this person open and ready to learn some behaviors, learn new coping skills? And, similarly, we need to assess the person's confidence in making the change and their self-efficacy level. Does she have a belief that she can accomplish these goals?

The H&B assessment areas that are of interest are **cognitive functioning** (very relevant to the rehab population), including orientation, awareness of limitations, executive functioning, attention, memory, comprehension, and judgment. What is the comprehension capacity, and ability to follow direction? Also, what is the level of frustration tolerance, and tolerance for ambiguity, and what type of behavioral controls are in place. All of these factors play a role in this person's participating in, and participating effectively, in his or her rehab. Tests include the Global Deterioration scale and Brief Cognitive Rating scale, the Cognistat, Montreal Cognitive Assessment scale, and the St. Louis University Mental Status scale.

Secondly, H&B assessment should include some measure of **psychological functioning**, in terms of anxiety and depression levels, as well as outlook and hopefulness. Third, the patient's **attitudes and motivation** are central to his or her response to treatment. We need to identify perseverance and persistence, and a belief in his or her ability to effect some change (i.e., self-efficacy). What is the person's understanding of this disability; how do they explain it to themselves. Are they accepting? Are they in denial? Some of these scales are the Geriatric Depression Scale, The Beck Hopeless Scale, Beck Depression Scale and Beck Depression Scale—Fast Screen, and the Dysfunctional Attitudes Scale of Medically Ill Elders.

The final assessment category is **coping strategy**. How effective are these coping strategies? Is the coping emotion-focused, that is, do they always react in an emotional way or is the usual coping style more problem-focused, where the person is learning ways to deal with these stresses in a more rational, non-emotional way. Tests for this category include Coping with Health Injuries and Problems, Illness Effects Questionnaire, the Patient Pain Profile, and the Rehabilitation Checklist.

It is highly recommended that the mental health practitioner keep handy a selection of these instruments in the test "briefcase" to have flexibility as to how the assessment progresses and what aspects of functioning are most in question.

The health and behavior "intervention" procedures are used to modify the psychological, behavioral, emotional, cognitive, and social factors identified as important to or directly affecting the patient's physiological functioning, disease status, health, and well-being. The focus of the intervention is to improve the patient's health and well-being, using cognitive, behavioral, social and/or psycho-physiological procedures designed to ameliorate specific disease-related problems. The major categories of interventions include psychoeducation, cognitive-behavioral therapy, skill development, anger and stress management, and support systems/family intervention.

The list below provides brief descriptions of the major interventions appropriate for these sessions.

**Anger Management** – teaching ways to monitor and change how events are perceived, how they are interpreted, and to learn what alternative responses are possible; anger management also requires the use of assertiveness training, relaxation training, and deep breathing to help reduce the intensity of the emotional response to the triggering event;

**Assertiveness Training** – evaluating communication patterns, differentiating among aggressive, passive, and assertive styles of communication; expressing feelings, desires, needs, and opinions constructively;

**Breathing Exercises** – increased awareness of breathing habits to use breathing as a relaxation skill, to release tension, and symptom release; deep breathing helps activate the part of the nervous system that controls relaxation; used to lower the level of stress-related arousal and tension;

**Coping Skills Training** – monitor effectiveness of denial, avoidance, regression, compensation, or rationalization, and the ability to convert unpleasant or unacceptable feelings and thoughts into more acceptable ones; educating and retraining patients to optimize the fit between stressors and applied coping strategies; identify non-adaptive cognitions and generate new possible solutions;

**Problem Solving Skills Training** – systematic approach to problems, and breaking down problems into smaller, more manageable ones that are solvable; developing a positive orientation toward the problem; confronting it and brainstorming possible solutions, goal setting and monitoring progress;

**Psychoeducation** – education about the role of anxiety and depression in chronic illness; role of thoughts and behaviors in emotional conditions; establish the link between health and behavioral health; how the behavioral health treatment fits into the overall interdisciplinary team approach;

**Relaxation Training** – progressive muscle relaxation to reduce physiological tension, and to create a state incompatible with anxiety by tensing and relaxing isolated muscle groups (legs, arms, shoulders, face/neck); helps to recognize difference between tension and relaxation;

**Self-Monitoring** – behavioral approach using detailed record keeping of targeted behavioral occurrences (day, time, activity, emotions) associated with behavior and efforts at self-regulation; useful in identifying maladaptive behavioral patterns targeted for change, then using problem solving and stimulus control techniques (i.e., identifying setting, people, internal or external events that are stimuli to behavior) to disrupt undesirable behavior patterns;

**Stimulus Control** – identifying situations, cues, or stimuli that trigger certain behaviors (positive or negative), and either promoting the exposure to these cues (for positive behavior) or reducing the exposure (for undesirable behaviors) to change the link between the cue and the behavior. For example, for weight loss programs, limiting the location where food is eaten is an example of stimulus control;

**Visualization** – Using mental pictures to induce relaxation; by bringing to mind images that are associated with relaxation, the autonomic arousal or tension is reduced.

### Documentation

I would be remiss if I did not discuss the real world aspects of psychotherapy with older adults, namely billing, documentation, and medical necessity. Medicare is an honor system, meaning that you provide services to your patient, you bill Medicare directly (or your agency does so, if you outsource billing), and you are paid by Medicare. They do not review your documentation. However, there is a look back period wherein Medicare has statutory authority of up to seven years after the fact when they can say "send all the documentation for beneficiary Mary Smith from the year 2001." Or, "Send documentation for these individual dates of service." That would be the first time they review your notes. Simply the fact that you have been paid for services all along does not mean that Medicare will never ask for your documentation. If they find services deemed to be medically unnecessary, even though they were paid seven years ago, they will ask for that money back. This is considered a "post-payment" Medical Review. Here are some essential points about billing and documentation:

1.  Each note must stand-alone. There must be a thread of continuity from the first encounter with the patient through each follow-up date of service. Each note standing alone means that services were medically necessary on each date, there is proof that the intervention could be provided only by a licensed mental health clinician, the patient evidenced adequate cognitive capacity for treatment, and there is definitive progress towards the goals and objectives.

2.  Content counts: no specific format is required. Content counts, not the structure. You may choose to use a SOAP note (subjective, objective, assessment, and plan) or a SIP note (status, intervention, and progress) or a DAP note (data or description, assessment, and plan)—any of those formats are fine. In fact, you may write a strictly narrative note if you prefer. A caveat about narratives: they may to be harder to follow without a structure. It's easier to inadvertently leave out data that you forgot to include, and the reviewer will have to search between the lines even harder. Some structure or format is therefore recommended to guarantee that you will meet each point in order to achieve medical necessity.

3.  Medicare defines individual psychotherapy as including work which is insight oriented, behavior modi-

fying, or supportive, or interactive insight, behavior modifying, or supportive work. A patient who has lost the ability to communicate verbally may use a language board, but interactive work is used more frequently with children. Medicare also covers group psychotherapy. Specific details are covered in the Carrier's "Local Coverage Determination" policy statements. Be cautious and explicit regarding the use of the term "supportive psychotherapy." It is required that you write more than "provided support." You must be using an intervention that requires a mental health practitioner such as yourself, not something that the nursing home staff can do.

There are five criteria for meeting medical necessity. The patient must meet all five criteria:

1. have a diagnosed mental disorder,
2. has active signs and symptoms of the disorder,
3. can engage in and benefit from psychotherapy,
4. interventions provided require a licensed mental health practitioner, and
5. is making reasonable, demonstrable progress.

All of these criteria apply to psychotherapy, whether provided individually or in groups. These five criteria place a high burden of proof on the psychotherapist, because each must be present on every note. Remember, every note must "stand alone." There are times when a Medicare payment denial has said that services might be *beneficial* to a patient, but not *medically necessary*. Unfortunately that usually is related to inadequate documentation, including statements such as "talked to the patient about her favorite TV show." While that may benefit the patient in terms of socialization and cognitive stimulation, it does not require a licensed mental health clinician, and it does not meet the five criteria.

Behavior medicine is reasonable and necessary according to these criteria:

1. the patient has an underlying illness or injury
2. the purpose of the treatment is not for treatment of a mental illness
3. the patient has adequate capacity to respond meaningfully
4. the specific interventions and outcomes have been clearly defined, and
5. the psychological intervention is required to address non-compliance with the medical treatment plan, or the biopsychosocial factors related to a newly diagnosed physical illness, or the exacerbation of an established illness.

It is also extremely important to establish the patient's cognitive appropriateness for participating and benefitting from treatment. The mental status is fairly easy to clarify: orientation to at least one person, and is able to retain concepts from session to session. It is also necessary to establish evidence that the patient is making progress toward the treatment goals and objectives. Thus, cognitive capacity and a willingness to work on identified problems and treatment objectives must be present.

In conclusion, there are numerous ways that psychologists can expand our roles as important members of the nursing home treatment team. We can raise the profile of mental or behavioral health services, explain how these services benefit patients and families, and can support and train caregivers in these settings. We can think about all the quick fixes that are available to our patients, especially like medication and other medical dictates, and how our profession can go beyond the quick fixes for more lasting benefit.

In a quote from a former chief justice of the Supreme Court, Oliver Wendell Holmes: *I would not give a fig for the simplicity this side of complexity, but I would give my life for the simplicity on the other side of complexity.*

# References

American Medical Association (2007). *Current Procedural Terminology*, Chicago, IL.

Blount, A. (1998). *Integrated Primary Care*, Norton, New York.

Camic, P. and Knight, S. (1998). *Clinical Handbook of Health Psychology*, Hogrefe & Huber, Kirkland, Washington.

Casciani, J.M. (2004). *The Practical Application of Health and Behavior Codes*, Annual Meeting of the American Psychological Association, Honolulu, HI.

Cummings, N., O'Donohue, W., and Ferguson, K. (2003). *Behavioral Health as Primary Care: Beyond Efficacy to Effectiveness*, Context Press, Reno, Nevada.

Cummings, N., O'Donohue, W., and Naylor, E. (2005). *Psychological Approaches to Chronic Disease Management*, Context Press, Reno, Nevada.

Falvo, D.R. (1999). *Medical and Psychosocial Aspects of Chronic Illness and Disability*, Aspen, Gaithersburg, Maryland.

Gatchel, R. and Oordt, M.S. (2003). *Clinical Health Psychology and Primary Care*, American Psychological Association, Washington D.C.

Haas, L.J. (2004). *Handbook of Primary Care Psychology*, Oxford, New York.

Hamberger, L.K., Ovide, C., and Weiner, E. (1999). *Making Collaborative Connections with Medical Providers*, Springer, New York.

Huber, C. and Backlund, B. (1996). *The Twenty Minute Counselor*, Crossroad, New York.

Hunter, C.L., Goodie, J.L., Oordt, M.S., and Dobmeyer, A.C. (2009). *Integrated Behavioral Health in Primary Care*, American Psychological Association, Washington, D.C.

Knight, R. (2001). *Psychotherapy with Older Adults.* Washington, DC: APA Books.

Kolbasovsky, A. (2008). *A Therapist's Guide to Understanding Common Medical Disorders*, Norton, New York.

Patterson, R. (2001). *Changing Patient Behavior*, Jossey Bass, San Francisco, California.

Patterson, J., Peek, C.J., Heinrich, R.L., Bischoff, R.J., and Scherger, J. (2002) *Mental Health Professionals in Medical Settings*, Norton, New York.

Rollnick, S., Mason, P., and Butler, C. (2000). *Health Behavior Change*, Harcourt, Edinburgh, UK.

Rosowsky, E., Casciani, J., and Arnold, M. (2009). *Geropsychology and Long Term Care: A Practitioner's Guide*, Springer, New York.

Sharoff, K. (2004). *Coping Skills Therapy for Managing Chronic and Terminal Illness*, Springer, New York.

Stuart, M. and Lieberman, J. (2002). *The Fifteen Minute Hour; Practical Therapeutic Interventions in Primary Care*, Saunders, Philadelphia.

Chapter 9

# Overmedicating America's Children: Medication and Alternatives to Treating ADHD

*(Edited from the transcript of the author's presentation)*

*William E. Pelham, Jr., Ph.D.*

What I'm going to talk about is the treatment for ADHD, but really I'm going to talk about whether or not we're focusing too much on medication for kids with ADHD, what the current standards are, and whether we should be thinking more in terms of using behavioral treatments as first-line treatment. So "Overmedicating America's Children" is the title I picked for my presentation, as it follows well those of the previous speakers.

I'm going to start first with disclosures, since I'm talking about drugs and that this laboratory and I have done a lot of work with pharmaceutical companies over the years. We helped develop many of the drugs that are now used with ADHD children. Thanks to Jim Swanson, I got involved in the Concerta studies. Jim did the original proof-of-concept work with Concerta and then expanded to include our group to do some of the first clinical trials comparing Concerta to standard methylphenidate. And we've done a lot of studies with Shire, Noven with the Daytrana patch, and a number of other pharmaceutical companies currently, along with psychiatrist Jim Maxmunski. We have a grant from Shire to look at medication for parents of ADHD children, when the parents also have ADHD, to look at whether medication for those parents helps the nature of their parent-child interactions. So we've done lots of work with pharmaceutical companies, and it's important to put disclosures up so the audience knows that we have had some relationships with these companies. I am not currently a consultant or scientific adviser or speaker for any of these companies.

The Center for Children and Families at Florida International University is growing. We are also in Buffalo and in Pittsburgh and with cooperating groups in a number of other locales and institutions.

So we're talking about ADHD that is characterized and has been for a very long time by three symptoms: inattention, hyperactivity, and impulsivity. For 50 years, those have been the core characteristics of ADHD. The debate in diagnosis has always been how many symptoms should be required and what combination of symptoms should be required to make that diagnosis, as these have changed in every Diagnostic and Statistical Manual (DSM). But I want to introduce the concept that I don't think we need to focus on symptoms if our goal is to figure out how to treat ADHD children. Instead, we should focus on impairment or problems in daily-life functioning. Impairment is explicit in the DSM in the sense that one must demonstrate impairment in real-life settings in order to make a diagnosis. Impairment is far more important than symptoms for a clinician. The reason for that is that kids don't get referred because of symptoms. So I've never had a mother come into a clinic or call on the telephone saying: Last night I was reading the DSM and I think my child has symptoms of ADHD. Instead, the mother calls and says: I'm calling you because my child's teacher told me yesterday at our annual teacher-parent conference that my child is being very disruptive in the classroom and she thinks he might have ADHD and said I need to go get an assessment or referral someplace. So that's why kids are referred. And actually Adrian Ingles has a big study, showing that in fact if you look at a very large level in mental health settings that's why kids get referred for mental health treatment, not because they have diagnoses, but because they have problems in daily-life functioning.

In addition, we have known for a long time that problems in daily-life functioning, and in key domains of daily-life functioning, is what predicts and mediates long-term outcome for children and adolescents who have mental health problems as they grow older. And the key domains are surprisingly consistent across a whole wide range of psychopathologies. Peer relationships, family factors (mainly parenting factors), and academic achievement or school problems are the three domains that seem to predict and to mediate long-term outcomes of a variety of types in children not only with ADHD, but other disruptive behavior disorders, learning disabilities, and so forth. So that means that assessment of impairment in daily-life functioning and assessment of adaptive skills is the most important thing we should focus on, not only in initial evaluation to determine what to treat, but in our ongoing assessments and evaluations of how the child is doing, because those are the domains that we need to change in order to improve the child currently and improve long-term outcomes.

So our goals for treatment of ADHD are not to normalize or minimize DSM symptoms, but to normalize or minimize impairments and to maximize adaptive functioning skills. That's the important thing to keep in mind. And that's a different view from the way most people approach psychopathology and ADHD.

So what is effective evidenced-based treatment for ADHD in children? There are lots of studies in ADHD. ADHD arguably has way more treatment outcome studies than most other forms of child psychopathology. There are two main treatments that have been used for decades: Central nervous system (CNS) stimulant medication, and behavioral modification. There are about twice as many studies of stimulant medication as there are of behavioral modification and they are larger studies, meaning both more studies and larger studies. And then there are a growing number of studies of a combination of those two, how you combine medication and psychosocial treatments? In general, the reviews and studies show that the effect sizes are moderate to large across a variety of treatments. The debates are: (a) do you get anything more if you combine the two treatments together than if you use them separately, and (b) which one should you use to start treatment first and so forth. But, in general, behavioral interventions and stimulant medication are by far the two most solidly evidence-based treatments for ADHD.

Now, one question that I want to focus on is: If you have two treatments both of which work, which one should you use as your first-line treatment? So what do you tell a family if they say, well, should I put my child on medication or should I try behavioral treatments first? So what do the professionals have to say about that? The American Academy of Pediatrics (AAP) guidelines for the treatment of ADHD say that the clinician should recommend either stimulant medication or behavioral therapy or the combination, and they don't specify a sequence. They just say either, or, or both.

In Japan, the guidelines for pediatricians say start with educational environmental adjustments. And that's really weak behavioral interventions. And then add behavioral treatment or medication or the combination after that.

The British National Health Service guidelines say start with behavioral parent training in the majority of cases and then add medication. And the guidelines say that, in most cases of moderate-to-severe ADHD, expect to add medication. So start with parent training, and for mild cases and some moderate cases, that should be sufficient.

The American Psychological Association (APA) Task Force on medications and psychosocial treatments in children published guidelines a couple years ago, saying that the decision about what treatment to use should be guided by the balance between benefits and harms. And, basically, that task force concluded, across the board for mental health disorders, there was evidence for the short-term effectiveness of medication, and evidence for the short-term effectiveness of psychosocial treatments, but the psychosocial treatments across the board had a lower risk of side effects. Therefore, you have two treatments, both of which appear to work about the same. If one has more side effects than the other, then in general you should start with the treatment that has fewer side effects. So that report recommends that in most cases of children, psychosocial interventions should be considered as the first line of treatment.

Now, in contrast, the American Academy of Child and Adolescent Psychiatry (AACAP) has current ADHD guidelines that say the first treatment should be medication, and if the first medication doesn't work of the dose you tried, and you tried different doses, then you try the second-line medication, and the third-line medication, and a fourth-line medication, and you try all of those prior to trying behavioral treatments. So behavioral treatments are listed as the fifth-line intervention for the treatment of ADHD, and they're equivalent to adding non-FDA-approved medications into the medications that you've tried that are not sufficient for the child.

So, again, you've got an APA saying, medication is the last thing you should use. You have the AAP saying, it doesn't matter which you start with; they're both good. And then you have the current AACAP guidelines that most child psychiatrists follow, saying, medication is the first thing that you should do. So there's quite a bit of controversy about which treatment you should be using first, and arguably what you use first is going to determine what the long-term course of the child's treatment is. So there's controversy here in the U.S. especially, and a lot of this resulted from a large federally-funded study, called "The MTA Collaborative Study" (Greenhill, Abikoff & Newcorn, 2000; Schafer, 2000). Our lab was a part of that when we were at the University of Pittsburgh prior to Buffalo. The MTA has been going on for a very long time. Actually, I can tell you how long because my son was born when the MTA was first funded and he just went off to college last month. So it's a long time, 18 years. But the MTA results, when they first came out, but not so much now, appeared to say that medication was to be the front-line treatment. I should also add that the eminent Dr. Swanson is also one of the investigators in the MTA, one of the original investigators in the MTA.

So what did the MTA results say when the first study was published, and what did the professional community say? This is a sampling of what people said when the first paper was published in 1999. With psychotropic medication as a front-line treatment, many children would not require behavioral interventions. Multimodal treatment offers little advantage over medication. The MTA study suggests there is very little benefit from any psychotherapeutic treatment.

I don't think most of those conclusions are warranted, but that's what most people were saying about the MTA results, and it extended beyond what people wrote about to what people said in reviews. This first paragraph is a review that a paper of ours got from Mina Dulcan, who was the editor of the *Journal of American Academy of Child & Adolescent Psychiatry* at the time. It referred to a drug study, but I have forgotten which drug study it was because we were publishing a lot of them in concert with pharmaceutical companies. It was one of the last paragraphs in the discussion in which we said that it's important to keep in mind that medication alone is not sufficient treatment for ADHD. One should always consider combining medication with psychosocial treatments. And she made us take that paragraph out because she said the MTA study didn't show that combined treatments were necessary.

Then a grant application reviewer for a grant for which we were applying said behavioral treatment and psychosocial intervention (such as parent training or school consultations), are rarely used in practice and unlikely to be used in the foreseeable future. So he recommended not funding our grant application.

So, again, there's a lot of controversy in the professional community about whether medication should be used, psychosocial treatment should be used, or they should be combined. And this is something that you don't see much if you are being trained to be a psychologist and believe in psychosocial treatments. But if you're working in the field of ADHD, who are you going to be working with for your entire career? They are the pediatricians and the psychiatrists who perform the other half of what goes on with children with ADHD. So you need to know about these medications and know what they're thinking, what their guidelines are in order to do an effective job in treatment.

There is a lot of money now being spent on medication as there are lots of kids taking medication. Most kids who take psychoactive drugs for their behavioral problems are kids who are taking ADHD medications. The Centers for Disease Control (CDC) came out with a review, and with a survey recently that showed that the biggest increase in all prescribed medications for adolescents over the last five years was actually stimulant medication for ADHD adolescents. And that comparison included all medications, not just psychoactive drugs. So the biggest increase in the whole medication field was for stimulant medication for ADHD adolescents. And the rates of the increase are pretty substantial.

These days in a doctor's office there seem to be drug company logos everywhere. As a parent, you start to realize this because when you go to your pediatrician and the pediatrician gives you the checklist that you're supposed to fill out about your child, even if it's just for a well-child visit, where you're writing down your information, the pen that you're using, the clipboard that you're using or the light that's on the table next to you, one of those is coming from a pharmaceutical company. So there's a big influence there. Who read the article in *The New York Times* recently about the chair of the Department of Psychiatry at Miami, Dr. Nemeroff? Nobody read that? As the article stated, there are a lot of people that are being castigated now for not revealing relationships with pharmaceutical companies and for having written things or done things in which they didn't make it clear that they were doing it on behalf of a pharmaceutical company.

Scheffler et al. (2007) report an enormous increase in medication use for ADHD from 1993 to 2003. There's been an increase by a factor of five in the use of medications over that decade and it didn't just happen in that decade. In the next four years, it continued to grow at the same rate, and according to the CDC, the increase of prescriptions has just continued to grow. It's not showing any signs of leveling off.

What do I think you need for comprehensive and effective treatment of ADHD? I don't think medication is the answer, even though it's the most widely used treatment and it's still increasing in the widespread nature of its use. I think it is behavioral parent training, school interventions, and when a child has severe peer problems, intensive peer interventions, and then medication should be used as an adjunctive treatment when it's needed. So that's my view of the way we should be doing medication for ADHD.

So why do I think that way? Well, one is that parent training, I believe, should be the backbone of treatment for ADHD kids, and it is absolutely central to affecting the long-term trajectory of these kids. A whole variety of parenting factors we know predict negative long-term outcomes in kids, and the presumption is that if we can change those, we can produce better outcomes in kids. Why is this the case? Why is parenting something that we need to change so much? Most people in this room who are parents realized when they became one that nobody ever taught you anything about being a parent. You have a child and after a day or two, then you have to go to the hospital and get your wife and baby to take them home, and you realize, then, you don't know anything. You simply don't know anything. You get home with a brand-new child that you don't know anything about what you're supposed to do. You know, you run to Barnes & Noble and you buy a little book called *In the First Year of Life*, right? Almost everybody who bought that little book then tries to figure it out from the book. But if you're on your own, you call your parents and ask them or your sister or your next-door neighbor. So nobody teaches us how to be parents, and it's the most important thing we do as a species, so we need to know more about parenting.

If you're a parent with an ADHD child born into the family, then you have a whole host of stressors and a child who is not going to be as responsive to traditional parenting approaches as most kids. So you need to be a better parent. You don't just need to learn how to be a good parent; you need to be a better parent than most people in order to handle your child with ADHD and maximize the chances of their having a good long-term outcome. ADHD children contribute dramatically to the parental stress and to disturbed parent-child relationships.

The parenting styles that are characteristic of ADHD parents are styles that we have known for a long time from developmental literature, and they predict the probability of long-term negative outcomes.

When I give talks to a room full of older adults, I like to ask, "How many of you are there in this room whose children have never caused you any stress? Raise your hands," and nobody raises their hand at all. And the reason for that is: parents know it's very stressful to have children. It's really stressful to have a child with ADHD. We did several studies early in my career where we showed that child behavioral problems actually cause parents to drink alcohol. And when parents drink alcohol it has a negative impact on the way they parent, and that negative parenting then worsens the child's behavior problems. So you get a vicious cycle going there. And these were very nice studies. They were laboratory investigations, where we actually manipulated child behavior, manipulated alcohol consumption, and demonstrated all of these connections. So the parenting part is a very important part of ADHD.

Why is it important to use behavioral treatments in school settings? We have known for years that ADHD children's primary problems occur in school. As bad as they are at home, they're worse in school. And teachers are no more equipped than parents to be dealing with children with ADHD. I have said for a long time, that teachers are given no training at all when they're in college about how to manage children with problematic behavior in school. They receive none whatsoever, even though such problematic behavior may be as high as 25% of the children in their classrooms. So we have to teach teachers that, because ADHD children have continuous and serious problems throughout their educational careers.

Why is it important to use behavioral treatments for peer relationship? I've already mentioned to you that ADHD kids have problems in those domains. Their problems with peers are well-established. We have known about them since Sue Campbell published a paper in 1977 or 1978, saying ADHD kids have problems with peers. So we need to work directly on their peer relationship problems. Also because peer relationships, many people believe, is the central mediator of long-term outcomes, that you need to change peer relationships in order to have a child that would have any hope of having a good outcome, especially for the most serious outcome domains, like peer relationships and criminal behavior.

So why do we treat ADHD in the summer program setting? It's because we can work on peer relationships in the summer program setting. It's very hard to work on this in any other kind of setting. You can do a little bit of it in school. You do nothing in a clinic. You can work on peer relationships in an intensive setting like a summer program, where it's ecologically valid. You have the kids playing games, doing the activities kids do regularly. You teach them skills in that context and provide ongoing supervision. You can teach competencies that the kids don't have. They can overcome some of their peer problems. Do you have an ADHD kid who's disruptive and aggressive with other kids or inattentive with other kids and impulsive with other kids? If you can make that child a good baseball player, that can go a long way toward his overcoming some of his problems, because, even if he's a pain in the ass, if he's good and he's going to be picked first when they're picking kids in teams, he'll feel good about that. He won't start the negative spiral that you could have and feelings of self-worth for ADHD kids by always being picked last in activities. So you can work on things that are adaptive skills and that are compensatory skills in this kind of setting.

So I mentioned briefly peer relationships, parent training, and school intervention. Stimulant medication is also an important component of treatment for some ADHD children, but I actually think it's a small minority of ADHD kids. I would bet that three-quarters to 80% of ADHD kids can be treated successfully without medication; and for the majority of the 29% or 25% that are left, it can be very low doses of medication, much lower than any doses anybody is using now. And low dose may be important in terms of minimizing side effects and maximizing the parents' parental and school involvement and treatment.

So I believe that medication should be initiated after you've started behavioral treatments, and you should try the evidence-based medications before cycling to other classes of drugs classes. I've seen very little research suggesting that any drugs other than the front-line stimulants, that are effective for ADHD. Even though it's very common for a psychiatrist to try stimulant one, stimulant two, stimulant three, and then switch to other classes of drugs, adding in other drugs or substituting other drugs, and the studies just aren't that good. There's not a lot reason to believe that if you add Risperdal and Clonidine to methylphenidate for treatment of a child with ADHD you're going to do anything other than increase the likelihood of side effects, even though it's the most common practice.

In addition, we have data that show that the minimal dose is what you should be thinking about, and the minimal dose, as I said, is much lower than what people typically prescribe. You don't need high doses of stimulants even when you need stimulants, especially if you start first with behavioral treatment, which is the point I'm making that we need to do.

And another consideration is that none of these drugs typically are things you can give for two weeks or six weeks and expect them to have any long-term effect. If they are going to be beneficial, they have to be continued for a long period of time, which makes the dose very important and makes the sequencing of treatments very important. That is, start with the behavioral and then add medication, because if you add medication first, you might undermine what the parents and the schools need to do. If you undermine that, then in the long run you're not going to have benefit.

How many people here have seen a child medicated with a stimulant? So if you've seen it, then you know all these things. The fastest way to get an ADHD child to behave better is to give him short-acting methylphenidate or just give the child regular old Dexedrine. If terrorist kidnapped me and took me to a foreign country because they had an ADHD child and they had heard that I could pick the treatment for ADHD, and they said, "Cure my child or we're going to shoot you," I would say, "Do you have access to methylphenidate around here?" This is because I know that it can make the child behave very well very quickly. I know it won't have any long-term benefit, but that person is not thinking five years ahead, and at least I would be released and out of captivity when the symptoms returned.

In any case, it's the fastest thing to do. It changes behavior very rapidly, which is one of the reasons why, I think it undermines parents' and teachers' willingness to do other treatments because it works very rapidly and it works very well in the short run and in a whole bunch of different outcomes measures, in the short run. But there are limitations to stimulant use, which are why we need to think about other approaches and, in my view, to emphasize other approaches being done first. I'll highlight just a couple.

Parents really aren't satisfied with medication as the sole form of treatment. When parents in the MTA study were asked which treatment they like the best and which one they would recommend to others, they recommended the behavioral treatment much more often than the medication and the combined treatment more than they chose medication. So medication was the least preferred treatment in the MTA study, even though some of the papers said the most effective treatment was medication and that was all you needed. That was not what the parents thought.

Papers have come out over the last 20 years that have failed to show that stimulants produce any long-term benefit. And the latest one is the one the MTA just published last year with Molina as the first author. This was the eight-year follow-up again showed no beneficial effect of stimulants. Dr. Swanson published the three-year follow-up that showed no beneficial effect of stimulants. And there are lots of other studies that have shown that.

You get that whether or not the studies were as well-defined or as well-designed as they could be, because the problem is that stimulants are widely available. So you can't have a randomized trial where half the kids get stimulants and half don't for five years, because anybody can get stimulants by going to their pediatrician and asking for them. So you're really looking at naturalistic longer-term studies. But people again in the more recent studies failed to show benefits in the long run.

Dr. Swanson has shown in the MTA study very elegantly, you get a reduction in growth with children in the MTA study, the only study that has these data, and that reduction in growth is, I would say, substantial. It's not five inches, as I was quoted as saying a number of years ago, but it's an inch, maybe two inches, and the point is that parents should be told that if they medicate their child and leave them on medication for five years, they will permanently lose an inch to two inches off their adult height.

And finally Jim and Nora Volkow have published a very important commentary, essentially saying that we just don't know much about the long-term safety of stimulant drugs. So, again, this goes back to what the APA said. If you have two treatments, and one of them is psychosocial and has arguably no physiological side effects, and the other one we don't know what the side effects are in the long run, but it's a treatment that directly affects the brain, that we might consider going with the less dangerous of the two treatments. Okay?

There are findings from our Concerta study: basically the medication dramatically helps functioning as regards classroom rule violations over the course of a very long day, but they didn't normalize it. So medication doesn't normalize things.

One of Steve Marcus's studies shows that over the course of a year under medicated database, the vast majority of children whose parents got a prescription for a stimulant drug, at day zero—that's when they got their prescription—and then they track who's still taking medication one year later. Almost nobody is still taking medication one year later. It just goes to the point that parents aren't satisfied with the treatment.

In the PALS follow-up study, we looked at stimulant use by grade, starting with children in grade one, and what it shows is that the peak year of stimulant use is grade four and then the kids stopped using medication after that. It declines a few kids every year until you get up to the point where they're eighteen or nineteen or twenty, very few people are still taking medication. No one told them to stop. The parents weren't made to stop; the kids weren't made to stop. But everybody stops medication over time. The MTA shows the same thing.

One of my concerns has also been that the way we medicate now, based on the MTA recommendations and current AA-CAP recommendations, is to use doses that are far higher than were used back in the 1980s and 1990s when most of the follow-up studies were conducted and published. Most of the studies on outcome and safety were done using an approach to medication that we're not using now. So I contrasted the two before 2000, which is when the MTA came out and Concerta and Adderall were approved. Most kids got medication for school hours only, which means they were medicated with short-acting medications. They just covered their behavior during school. They didn't get medication on weekends. They didn't get medication in the summer. The typical dose for a methylphenidate equivalence was 15–20 mg a day, and most kids were medicated for one to three years. So if you just take those numbers and do a little hypothetical experiment, you can compute how much medication a typical child would take in its lifetime. It's five to ten thousand mg of methylphenidate. After the MTA came out saying that higher doses were necessary and the kids should take medication seven days a week, 365 days a year, and after the two long-acting medications came out that presumed the kids were going to take medication all day long because that's the nature of the pill. You take Concerta or Adderall first thing in the morning, it lasts for 12 hours. So you're medicated all day long. So if in a hypothetical experiment you take the current recommendations to start medication early, as the MTA recommended, and continue as long as necessary, continue all the way through the school years and 365 days a year instead of half the days of the year and just using the same dose equivalent of Concerta and Adderall XR, you're giving a third more medication every day. This is almost 80% more medication every day just because of the formulation. So then you use that to compute a lifetime dose; and you end up with a far higher number. And then you ask, is 175,000 mg of methylphenidate in a lifetime safe compared to 7,500 mg? And the answer is: We don't know. We don't know whether it's safe or not, but this is the current approach to medication that is recommended in the guidelines for the American Academy of Child & Adolescent Psychiatry.

So, in summary, these are the four treatments that are used to treat ADHD. Parent training and school intervention are what you should always be doing. I argue you should start with it. I say, child intervention use when needed, because I don't believe that social skills training that is clinic-based is effective. And to have effective peer-based treatment, you need to do much more intensive interventions like summer treatment programs (STPs). If you don't need a really expensive treatment, we shouldn't be providing a really expensive treatment. So I think you use that when you need it based on peer problems. And also you should use medication only when you need it. It means, after you've tried everything else, try medication if you need it.

Summarizing the results of the MTA study, it is like the blind man and the elephant. What does that creature look like? Depending on what each blind person touched, they thought the elephant was shaped like that. So depending on whom you are and how you look at it, the MTA results mean very different things to different people.

The basic finding of the MTA study is best summarized thus: The two medication groups in the MTA got better. The treatment lasted one year. So they were better at the end of treatment. And then over the next year and then over the next two years and then the next five years, the treatment differences all disappear. So the original recommendation of the MTA study was all based on the first year result. And if you look at results down the line, it doesn't look like medication actually was differentially beneficial for the children. But this is a very influential study that really affected all of these guidelines that I've talked to you about and probably, arguably was the cause of the dramatic increase in medication dosing.

Except, I have to say that there is one limitation of that. Looking at the long-term dosing effects, I was surprised, because the difference in dosing between people in the behavioral treatment and in people who started in the medication treatment, it wasn't that great. Well, most of the behavioral people, or at least many of the behavioral-treated subjects never got medication. The parents left them off medication for a long time. So we were looking at the numbers to try to figure out why they were so much more similar at follow-up than when they started off. And actually it looks like what happened is, in the year 2000, the dosing for the kids in that group all shot up dramatically. And what would that mean? What happened in the year 2000? What drugs became available? They were Concerta and Adderall XR. So the doctors for all those kids who had been taking short-acting methylphenidate for school days only now got switched by their doctors to Concerta and Adderall XR and their doses skyrocketed. So after that point, the doses for all the groups look more similar, and that was the shift caused by the introduction of two new medications to the psychopharmacology armamentarium.

So let's me just say that the MTA answered a lot of questions, but left a lot of questions unanswered. So it doesn't tell us what treatment the child needs. It tells us, if a child is randomly assigned to four treatments, which one will produce relatively better outcomes, but not for the child standing in front of you. What treatment does *this* child need? It doesn't tell you anything about sequencing. We had many discussions in the course of the MTA in the year it took us to design the study about sequencing. Should we start treatment simultaneously in the combined group? Should the combined people get medication before they start the behavioral treatment or the opposite, or should they both start at the same point in time? And what we ended up doing was starting everybody at the same point in time. So both of the treatments got started together. It doesn't tell us what the best doses of treatment are, because in the MTA everybody got the same dose. They got whatever we designed was the dose of treatment, which was intensive medication and intensive behavioral treatment. The MTA didn't say anything about what starts first and what starts second and whether you should combine treatments or whether you should start with low-intensity behavioral treatments and then move to high-intensity behavioral treatments if the low intensity didn't work, instead of adding medication. So it didn't address any of those questions. It didn't talk about implications of different doses and sequences for benefit and risk of side effects. And the reason that these are important issues is that this is what you as a clinician have to think about every day. It's what an ADHD child's pediatrician has to think about. Okay. I've a kid in front of me.

What should I do? What should I start with? I've got a bunch of drugs. I've got parent training maybe. If you're a pediatrician, you have to find somebody who does parent training and then figure out how to get the parent to them. If you're a psychologist, you have to find a pediatrician who will do the medication in conjunction, working with you. So you have to find people to do it and you have to decide what you're going to do.

So these are the questions that a practitioner has to decide on a daily basis and that families have to decide also. So this is what we've been working on this lab for the last decade, looking at the answers to some of these treatments, all of which grew out of our experience in the MTA study.

So this is the first study and the second—actually the third study that we did in the sequence of studies. There was a large one where we looked at medication and behavioral treatment and the combination of the two at different dosage levels. We've done a lot of studies and a lot of people have done studies, including Dr. Swanson. They looked at dose of medication, but nobody had ever done a study looking at dose of behavioral therapy. Do you need a high dose or a low dose of behavior therapy if you're treating kids? And does your need change depending on whether the child is taking medication and vice versa? Does the dose of medication change as a function of whether you're getting any behavioral treatment, and, if so, how much? So we designed the study in the context of the STP, where you got if you were a child in the summer treatment program, you either got: (a) high-intensity behavioral modification (B-mod), the definition of which was our regular treatment in the summer program, or (b) you got no behavioral modification. And what that meant was, we took away all of our treatment. The kids still had to come there every day. The staff still had to interact with them. But they were prohibited from using behavioral interventions with the kids. This meant you couldn't put kids in time-out; you couldn't use points with them;

you couldn't send a daily report card home telling the parents how they had done; you couldn't do any behavioral interventions. And I do remember describing this once to a pharmaceutical company rep, who said, "Well, that's a ridiculous study because real life isn't like that at all." And I said, "I know, because in real life everybody uses behavior modification all the time." So if you're doing a study you actually have to have a controlled setting like this to demonstrate what the difference is between no behavior modification and some behavior modification, because you can't find a classroom in the country where a teacher doesn't use behavioral modification routinely.

The no B-mod days were very difficult. The only fallback intervention was, we had a suspension room. If the kid was too bad, he was dangerous to other kids, he was picking up rocks and throwing them at the other kids in the group, we had to remove him from the group, and then he went to a suspension room. And the suspension rooms were manned by the staff in the program. Anyway, what that meant is, you had to keep the kid in the room until the staff decided that it was okay to put him back in the group. Sometimes that was ten minutes and sometimes it was an hour, depending on whether you thought the child had calmed down and so forth. And we didn't want to do that. We didn't plan to do that. But we realized pretty quickly in the study we had to have some contingency like that for when children got completely out of control.

And then the low-intensity behavioral modification was to say, can we take our behavior treatments and water them down enough so that they can be done in a non-intensive setting and therefore would cost less? It would be less complicated to implement. So in the STP classroom, it was an intervention that we thought we could have the regular classroom teachers to implement. You wouldn't need a special education teacher and lots of aides to do it. Any teacher could do it. And what that meant was, we took out the most complicated part of the STP, which is the point system, where you're earning points for good behaviors, losing them for bad behaviors, and you're getting told constantly how you're doing with earning and losing points. That's the backbone of the intervention. And we took that out. So we still had daily report cards. We still had lots of praise going on the part of the staff. But we took out the point system. And that is arguably the most complex and thus the most expensive part of the treatment. If you don't have to have highly trained staff to implement a point system, you don't need to have as many people in an STP staffing it; therefore, it won't cost as much.

Then we crossed those three treatments with four different doses of medication: (a) no medication, (b) placebo, (c) the standard doses that were used in most dosing studies of ADHD, 0.3 and 0.6 mg/kg/dose, and (d) then a half dose. So we used less than 0.3 mg/kg—0.15 mg/kg. And we did this because we had done a pilot study that to our surprise showed that particular dose of medication had a very large effect on kids. It's a dose that people weren't using in studies. It was used in two studies in the previous 30 years: One Bob Sprague did many years ago and one actually I did many years ago and then I forgot that I did it. Anyway, so we crossed these four treatments. In STP studies, the way the medication is manipulated is, you change the dose every day, because with stimulant drugs, they take effect right away, they wear off right away, each day is a new day. So you randomize the dose over days; therefore, taking a huge advantage, because you have randomization of doses over days. The behavioral treatment was counter-balanced. So it couldn't be randomized by kid, because we have all these kids in groups together. So a whole group got no B-mod for three weeks or low B-mod for three weeks or high B-mod for three weeks, with the order of those counter-balanced across the groups. So you have three weeks of no B-mod and you're going on and off medication in different doses during those three weeks if you're an individual child, and each child's medication dosing regimen is different from every other child's or independent of every other child's. They are all randomly determined. So that's an example.

A typical finding from the first year of the study from classroom rule violations, sixty rule violations in thirty minutes was probably about what you got. Right? And that's sixty rule violations per child. So you multiply that by twelve and you had 700 rule violations occurring in a thirty-minute period. I have a nice picture, actually, of Greg Fabiano standing next to a point board with a teacher, and the point board was a white board in the beginning of the day; it was black by the end of the 30-minute period because they had so many small marks on it.

Anyway, that shows a couple of surprising things. One, it shows a very clear linear effect of methylphenidate. Right? And it shows that that a low dose had some effect. We didn't think it would have a big effect, but it had some effect. You double the dose, you get a bigger effect. You double the dose again, you get a bigger effect. Now, we also have data points reflecting what normal kids are like in the STP, because for this study we had normal kids that we recruited and we sprinkled them into the STP groups. They didn't get medication, but they got everything else that the kids got. We wanted that so we could see what normalization was like, what normal kids behaved like and how close we could get to that. So, if you don't have any behavioral modification going on you need a fairly high dose of medication to get good functioning, to get anywhere close to the level of the normal kids, 0.6 mg/kg, because you don't get there with 0.3 mg/kg. And this is important, because we published years of studies in the STP, where we're doing medication studies that were just lying on top of our behavioral intervention as a background that showed that you got really big effects at 0.3 mg/kg and it topped off. We didn't get much bigger effect by doubling the dose. Well, this shows that actually this was because we were only looking at these conditions in all of our previous studies because we've never had a no B-mod condition. So that validates what you can show if you have a condition where you have no behavioral modification at all going on.

The second point is that it shows very clearly, if you look at just the placebo column, the difference between no B-mod and B-mod days is enormous. So you go from sixty rule violations per thirty minutes, or one hundred twenty-five per hour rate, down to between seven and fifteen, depending on your condition. And that's a huge drop. And that drop is bigger than the drop you see with medication. So the effects of behavioral modification are at least as good, and maybe even larger, than medication if you do a study where you're really controlling very tightly the medication and the behavioral modification. So this is an interesting study because it says that it is not the case that in a head-to-head comparison medication always wins. If you design a study so you have a true no behavioral modification condition and true no medication condition and you manipulate doses, then you can show behavioral treatment is as bad or as good as medication in a controlled setting.

The third point I want to make is that those medication lines, the medication dose lines, when you have behavioral treatment as the background, are almost flat. This shows a clear linear effect of medication: the more medication, you get better. But there is a point at which you get almost nothing when you double the dose of medication or when you double the dose of medication again. So if you use behavioral intervention, this suggests that if you're using behavioral intervention as your first-line treatment, maybe you can use tiny doses of medication, like 0.15 mg/kg if some kids need it. It looks like a lot of kids might do fine without it. But if they need it, maybe you can use a tiny dose and get away with a really low dose of medication and not have to use a higher dose that causes side effects. And in this study, no child, not one child, out of the one hundred fifty kids in the study had a single side effect rated by a parent or a teacher or a counselor at the low-dose of medication. Not one child had one side effect rated. All the side effects started at 0.3 mg/kg, and they got a lot higher at 0.6 mg/kg.

So, again, this suggests that if you're going to use medication, low doses, in conjunction with behavioral therapy, might max out your additional benefit and cause no side effects. Jim Maxmunski has looked at this for the follow-up children in the study, and at .15 mg/kg, kids who stayed on that dose in follow-up didn't have any weight loss and didn't have any gross depression, as they did in the MTA. So, again, it says that low medications may be important, but what this shows also is that a low dose of medications alone is not going to be anywhere near normalized functioning. It's low medication in conjunction with behavioral treatment that gets you down into that good range.

So this is a follow-up—there were three studies that were the follow-up to the study I just showed you. We're still analyzing data and then writing them up. In an adaptive study, which we just finished last year, we looked at the question of dose and of sequencing. Is it better to start with medication or is it better to start with behavioral modification? In the previous study, we controlled everything. Everybody got all the treatments; they all started at the same time, stopped at the same time, so forth. So this study was done in regular school setting. Here, we're looking at whether it makes a difference what treatment you start with, and then if a child is nonresponsive or insufficiently responsive to what you started with, what should you do? Should you double the dose of what you started with or should you add any other modality? Those kids started random assignment at the start and a low dose of medication or a low dose of behavior modification. A low dose of medication was 0.15 mg/kg twice a day at school. The low dose of behavior modification was eight sessions of group parent training and a teacher daily report card, a consultation from a staff member to go and set up a daily report card with a teacher. And that was the intervention.

After eight weeks of intervention, we assessed at the eight-week point how kids were doing. We used two measures to see how kids were doing. If they were doing fine, if their teacher said they were doing fine, then they just stayed in that treatment arm, which meant they continued to get medication and the teacher just continued to implement a daily report card. We didn't have more consultation coming from the staff member; the teacher just continued to implement the daily report card. If they were fine on the medication, they just continued to get the same dose of medication. If they were not doing as well as our predefined levels indicated, then they were re-randomized. So if you were doing well after this, you just stayed in the treatment arm. If you're not doing well, you got re-randomized. And the re-randomization was either to add the other modality or intensify the dose of what you started with. So if you were a kid who was assigned to B-mod and you weren't doing well, then you got assigned to get more B-mod. And what you got depended on the team of professionals' decisions and on your areas of impairment. And you can have basically anything. You could have an aide come into the classroom. You could have more parent training sessions. You could have a variety of things.

And if you're in the medication condition and you weren't doing as well as necessary, then you got a higher dose of medication. And the study separated school and home, so the functioning at school was rated by the teacher; functioning at home was rated by your parent. And the decisions about going up or down were independent.

By the end of the school year, almost all the kids were re-randomized. In the school setting, 56% of the med-first kids stayed on the medication and 36% of the B-mod first just stayed on regular B-mod. So two-thirds of B-mod kids needed to be re-randomized at school and 44% of the medication kids needed to be re-randomized in the school. There were a couple of surprising points in that. One is that 44% of the kids who were given 0.15 mg/kg methylphenidate in school and that's all they got, did fine the entire school year. I was flabbergasted with that result, as was Jim Maxmunski, who was the psychiatrist who was thinking nobody is going to survive on that dose of medication.

The second is that, on a very low dose of behavior modification, just one set of contacts with a teacher to set up the daily report card, a third of the kids were fine for the rest of that year.

As for the home situation, there was much more randomization, and there were some interesting parts about that. So the most interesting question was for us, which of these different sequences and which of these treatments was the most effective? Overall, which one is most effective? You have to analyze is the three groups versus three other groups. So you're putting all the kids in these three groups together at the end and comparing them to these three groups. You can do some post hoc observation, or analyses to compare groups within treatments, and compare groups across treatments. What the results showed are the direct observations in the classroom by independent observers that showed getting behavior modification first caused better behavior at school at the end of the year. There were substantial differences in classroom functioning. Even though this is secondary-level analyses because what it shows is that obviously if you're medication is not re-randomized and behavior-first is not re-randomized, you're going to be better than anybody else by definition, because you weren't bad at the eight-week point. So you never got re-randomized. But if you were looking at which is better—if somebody is going to end up in multimodal treatment—that is, they're getting both medication and behavioral treatment, which one works best?

Well, looking at people who got medication first and then had behavioral treatment added, and looking at who got behavioral treatment first and had medication added in, lower is better. So what that shows is that multimodal treatment is more effective if you start with the behavioral treatment. If you're going to end up with multimodal treatment, it's more effective if you start with behavioral treatment and also—again to my surprise, people who started with behavioral treatment and got re-randomized to behavioral treatment are doing better than people who started on medication and got re-randomized to medication.

So this is a very interesting study, because it makes behavioral treatment and the importance of starting with it, look very good compared to some of the big randomized trials like the MTA. Now, why might that happen? Why might starting with behavioral treatment be better? One possible answer is that if you started your low-dose treatment with eight parent training sessions and a school consultation versus if you started your treatment with medication and you didn't do well and then you were re-randomized to start attending parent training, far fewer people came to the parent training than did if they were first started with behavior modification.

What you see is that if you were medication first versus B-mod first, only 40% of those people even attended one parent training session. And if you look at adequate dose of parent training, defined as 75%, 70% of the behavioral-treatment-first group got 75% of the parent training sessions—that is, they came to parent training—and that was true for only 15% of the combined group.

So we think this may contribute to the results that I showed you. Maybe the active ingredient in why kids don't do as well is that their parents don't get the treatment, as they elect not to come in. Now, why did they elect not to come in? Maybe they're satisfied with the way their kids are behaving if they get medication. So they don't feel the need to come in. That can't be entirely the story, because, remember, the only people who got assigned to get more treatment were people whose kids weren't doing as well as we would have liked. But it may be only a part of the story. It would be nice if we had information about what the teachers were doing in the classroom. Actually, we do have observations of it, but we don't have the same kind of intervention because, to do this study, we had to set up the equivalent to daily report cards in the classes of all the kids. Even if they weren't in a behavioral treatment, we set up a faux daily report card. So the teachers picked target behaviors, they evaluated them, and that was one of the variables that we were using to define a positive response for kids. Because it was a measure in the study, we had to make sure it got done. So even for kids in the medication group, the therapist contacted the teachers, making sure they filled out that little form every day. The kid didn't know anything about the form. The parents didn't know anything about the form. But it was the same kind of form. So we don't have a good sense of whether teachers were doing things like parents did, because we essentially forced teachers to do the daily report cards every day, because they were an important part of the study.

But I think what this suggests is that medication really undermines parents' willingness to get involved in treatment. That's one of the major outcomes of this study. The sequence of starting with behavioral first and then adding medication works better than starting with medication and then adding behavioral treatment, arguably because it undermines parental motivation. That was true even for the booster sessions. I forgot to mention that. After the first eight weeks, parents had the option of coming once a month to a group booster session. And you can see the difference in attendance at the booster sessions also is a function of sequence of treatments.

## Conclusions

What conclusions can we draw from this series of studies? I've skipped one of the studies, but over the years of doing these treatments, we had six cohorts of people that received the treatment for a year. Three hundred families of one cohort got three years of treatment in one of the studies I skipped. So we had almost five hundred families over that seven-year span where we were doing intensive parent training, STPs, school-based interventions, and so forth, a tremendous effort on the part of the staff who had recruited all those kids and to run it through all the studies. What they showed is that dose of treatment is important, especially in comparative studies. If you want to minimize the amount of medication you take, or if you want to keep the dose of medication low, then start your treatment with the behavioral treatment and you don't need as much medication per kid.

At high doses of either treatment, there's no additive value of it. So you'd have to go back to what we looked at in the beginning about classroom rule violations and think about that. What we saw was that, if you had high dose of behavioral modification, then you got almost nothing by adding medication into that. And if you had a high dose of medication, you got almost nothing by adding behavioral treatment into it. And the MTA study used a high dose of both treatments, and that may be one reason why the MTA combined treatment condition wasn't that much better than medication. What this shows is that if you manipulate dose, you can produce that effect. Under optimal conditions, the two treatments have comparable effects and limitations and sequencing treatments is important.

# References

Greenhill, Abikoff & Newcorn (2000). Multimodal treatment of ADHD offers little advantage over medication. *Journal of the American Academy of Child and Adolescent Psychiatry,* 23, 110-122.

MTACG (1999). The MTA study. *National Institute of Mental Health,* Washington, DC.

Shaffer, D. (2000). MTA studies suggest very little benefit from any psychotherapeutic treatment. *Journal of the American Academy of Child and Adolescent Psychiatry,* 23, 124-143.

Scheffler, R.M., Hinshaw, S.P., Modrek, S., & Levine, P. (2007). Trends: The global market for ADHD medications. *Affairs,* 28(2). 480-487.

Note: Most of the studies referred to by the author and not cited in detail are those in which Dr. Pelham is the lead author. Complete references may be obtained by contacting Dr. Pelham at Florida International University.